Health & Fitness

Editor: Tracy Biram

Volume 384

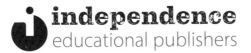
independence
educational publishers

First published by Independence Educational Publishers

The Studio, High Green

Great Shelford

Cambridge CB22 5EG

England

© Independence 2021

Copyright

Photocopy licence

ISBN-13: 978 1 86168 842 2

Printed in Great Britain

Zenith Print Group

Contents

Introduction

Health & Fitness is Volume 384 in the **issues** series. The aim of the series is to offer current, diverse information about important issues in our world, from a UK perspective.

ABOUT HEALTH & FITNESS

Across the world, obesity has nearly tripled since 1975. This book explores the reasons behind the rise in weight, and looks at how we can tackle the obesity crisis. With our lifestyles becoming increasingly sedentary, we all need to be more active, but just how active should we be? We also look at the link between physical activity and mental health. From PE at school, to participation in sport in later life, being active has so many benefits, including helping us to lead a healthy lifestyle.

OUR SOURCES

Titles in the **issues** series are designed to function as educational resource books, providing a balanced overview of a specific subject.

The information in our books is comprised of facts, articles and opinions from many different sources, including:

♦ Newspaper reports and opinion pieces

♦ Website factsheets

♦ Magazine and journal articles

♦ Statistics and surveys

♦ Government reports

♦ Literature from special interest groups.

A NOTE ON CRITICAL EVALUATION

Because the information reprinted here is from a number of different sources, readers should bear in mind the origin of the text and whether the source is likely to have a particular bias when presenting information (or when conducting their research). It is hoped that, as you read about the many aspects of the issues explored in this book, you will critically evaluate the information presented.

It is important that you decide whether you are being presented with facts or opinions. Does the writer give a biased or unbiased report? If an opinion is being expressed, do you agree with the writer? Is there potential bias to the 'facts' or statistics behind an article?

ASSIGNMENTS

In the back of this book, you will find a selection of assignments designed to help you engage with the articles you have been reading and to explore your own opinions. Some tasks will take longer than others and there is a mixture of design, writing and research-based activities that you can complete alone or in a group.

FURTHER RESEARCH

At the end of each article we have listed its source and a website that you can visit if you would like to conduct your own research. Please remember to critically evaluate any sources that you consult and consider whether the information you are viewing is accurate and unbiased.

Useful Websites

www.digital.nhs.uk

www.eufic.org

www.gov.uk

www.hcmmag.com

www.independent.co.uk

www.netdoctor.co.uk

www.nhs.uk

www.obesityhealthalliance.org.uk

www.psychologytoday.com

www.publichealthmatters.blog.gov.uk

www.raceatyourpace.co.uk

www.reading.ac.uk

www.sportengland.org

www.telegraph.co.uk

www.theconversation.com

www.thelancet.com

www.ucl.ac.uk

www.wellbeingpeople.com

www.who.int

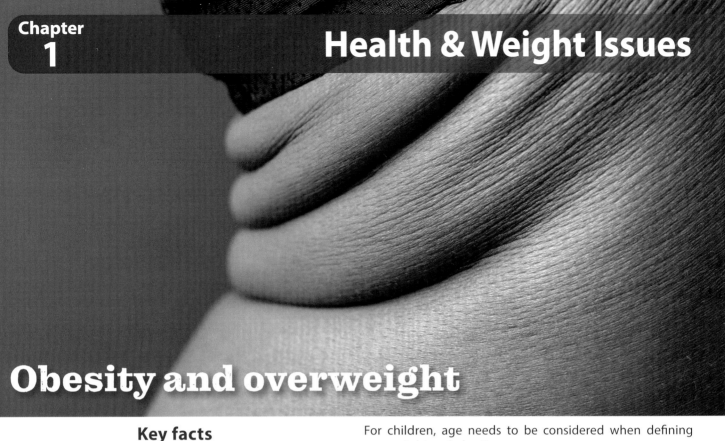

Obesity and overweight

Key facts

♦ Worldwide obesity has nearly tripled since 1975.

♦ In 2016, more than 1.9 billion adults, 18 years and older, were overweight. Of these over 650 million were obese.

♦ 39% of adults aged 18 years and over were overweight in 2016, and 13% were obese.

♦ Most of the world's population live in countries where overweight and obesity kills more people than underweight.

♦ 38 million children under the age of 5 were overweight or obese in 2019.

♦ Over 340 million children and adolescents aged 5-19 were overweight or obese in 2016.

♦ Obesity is preventable.

What are obesity and overweight?

Overweight and obesity are defined as abnormal or excessive fat accumulation that may impair health.

Body mass index (BMI) is a simple index of weight-for-height that is commonly used to classify overweight and obesity in adults. It is defined as a person's weight in kilograms divided by the square of his height in meters (kg/m2).

Adults

For adults, WHO defines overweight and obesity as follows:

♦ overweight is a BMI greater than or equal to 25; and

♦ obesity is a BMI greater than or equal to 30.

BMI provides the most useful population-level measure of overweight and obesity as it is the same for both sexes and for all ages of adults. However, it should be considered a rough guide because it may not correspond to the same degree of fatness in different individuals.

For children, age needs to be considered when defining overweight and obesity.

Children under 5 years of age

For children under 5 years of age:

♦ overweight is weight-for-height greater than 2 standard deviations above WHO Child Growth Standards median; and

♦ obesity is weight-for-height greater than 3 standard deviations above the WHO Child Growth Standards median.

Children aged between 5–19 years

Overweight and obesity are defined as follows for children aged between 5–19 years:

♦ overweight is BMI-for-age greater than 1 standard deviation above the WHO Growth Reference median; and

♦ obesity is greater than 2 standard deviations above the WHO Growth Reference median.

Facts about overweight and obesity

Some recent WHO global estimates follow.

In 2016, more than 1.9 billion adults aged 18 years and older were overweight. Of these over 650 million adults were obese.

♦ In 2016, 39% of adults aged 18 years and over (39% of men and 40% of women) were overweight.

♦ Overall, about 13% of the world's adult population (11% of men and 15% of women) were obese in 2016.

♦ The worldwide prevalence of obesity nearly tripled between 1975 and 2016.

♦ In 2019, an estimated 38.2 million children under the age of 5 years were overweight or obese. Once considered a high-income country problem, overweight and obesity are now on the rise in low- and middle-income countries, particularly in urban settings. In Africa, the number of overweight children under 5 has increased by nearly 24% since 2000. Almost half of the children under 5 who were overweight or obese in 2019 lived in Asia.

Over 340 million children and adolescents aged 5-19 were overweight or obese in 2016.

The prevalence of overweight and obesity among children and adolescents aged 5-19 has risen dramatically from just 4% in 1975 to just over 18% in 2016. The rise has occurred similarly among both boys and girls: in 2016 18% of girls and 19% of boys were overweight.

While just under 1% of children and adolescents aged 5-19 were obese in 1975, more than 124 million children and adolescents (6% of girls and 8% of boys) were obese in 2016.

Overweight and obesity are linked to more deaths worldwide than underweight. Globally there are more people who are obese than underweight – this occurs in every region except parts of sub-Saharan Africa and Asia.

What causes obesity and overweight?

The fundamental cause of obesity and overweight is an energy imbalance between calories consumed and calories expended. Globally, there has been:

♦ an increased intake of energy-dense foods that are high in fat and sugars; and

♦ an increase in physical inactivity due to the increasingly sedentary nature of many forms of work, changing modes of transportation, and increasing urbanization.

Changes in dietary and physical activity patterns are often the result of environmental and societal changes associated with development and lack of supportive policies in sectors such as health, agriculture, transport, urban planning, environment, food processing, distribution, marketing, and education.

What are common health consequences of overweight and obesity?

Raised BMI is a major risk factor for noncommunicable diseases such as:

♦ cardiovascular diseases (mainly heart disease and stroke), which were the leading cause of death in 2012;

♦ diabetes;

♦ musculoskeletal disorders (especially osteoarthritis – a highly disabling degenerative disease of the joints);

♦ some cancers (including endometrial, breast, ovarian, prostate, liver, gallbladder, kidney, and colon).

The risk for these noncommunicable diseases increases, with increases in BMI.

Childhood obesity is associated with a higher chance of obesity, premature death and disability in adulthood. But in addition to increased future risks, obese children experience breathing difficulties, increased risk of fractures, hypertension, early markers of cardiovascular disease, insulin resistance and psychological effects.

Facing a double burden of malnutrition

Many low- and middle-income countries are now facing a 'double burden' of malnutrition.

While these countries continue to deal with the problems of infectious diseases and undernutrition, they are also experiencing a rapid upsurge in noncommunicable disease risk factors such as obesity and overweight, particularly in urban settings.

It is not uncommon to find undernutrition and obesity co-existing within the same country, the same community and the same household.

Children in low- and middle-income countries are more vulnerable to inadequate pre-natal, infant, and young child nutrition. At the same time, these children are exposed to high-fat, high-sugar, high-salt, energy-dense, and

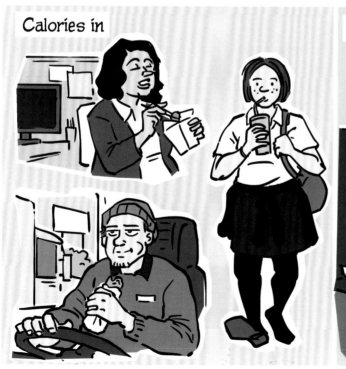

Calories in

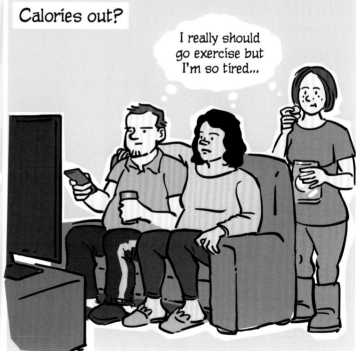

Calories out?

I really should go exercise but I'm so tired...

micronutrient-poor foods, which tend to be lower in cost but also lower in nutrient quality. These dietary patterns, in conjunction with lower levels of physical activity, result in sharp increases in childhood obesity while undernutrition issues remain unsolved.

How can overweight and obesity be reduced?

Overweight and obesity, as well as their related noncommunicable diseases, are largely preventable. Supportive environments and communities are fundamental in shaping people's choices, by making the choice of healthier foods and regular physical activity the easiest choice (the choice that is the most accessible, available and affordable), and therefore preventing overweight and obesity.

At the individual level, people can:

◆ limit energy intake from total fats and sugars;

◆ increase consumption of fruit and vegetables, as well as legumes, whole grains and nuts; and

◆ engage in regular physical activity (60 minutes a day for children and 150 minutes spread through the week for adults).

Individual responsibility can only have its full effect where people have access to a healthy lifestyle. Therefore, at the societal level it is important to support individuals in following the recommendations above, through sustained implementation of evidence based and population based policies that make regular physical activity and healthier dietary choices available, affordable and easily accessible to everyone, particularly to the poorest individuals. An example of such a policy is a tax on sugar sweetened beverages.

The food industry can play a significant role in promoting healthy diets by:

◆ reducing the fat, sugar and salt content of processed foods;

◆ ensuring that healthy and nutritious choices are available and affordable to all consumers;

◆ restricting marketing of foods high in sugars, salt and fats, especially those foods aimed at children and teenagers; and

◆ ensuring the availability of healthy food choices and supporting regular physical activity practice in the workplace.

WHO response

Adopted by the World Health Assembly in 2004 and recognized again in a 2011 political declaration on noncommunicable disease (NCDs), the 'WHO Global Strategy on Diet, Physical Activity and Health' describes the actions needed to support healthy diets and regular physical activity. The Strategy calls upon all stakeholders to take action at global, regional and local levels to improve diets and physical activity patterns at the population level.

The 2030 Agenda for Sustainable Development recognizes NCDs as a major challenge for sustainable development. As part of the Agenda, Heads of State and Government committed to develop ambitious national responses, by

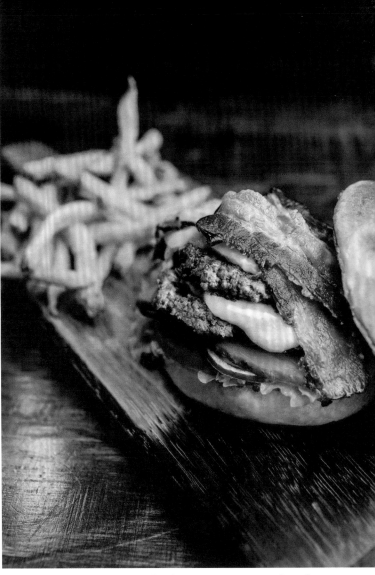

2030, to reduce by one-third premature mortality from NCDs through prevention and treatment (SDG target 3.4).

The 'Global action plan on physical activity 2018–2030: more active people for a healthier world' provides effective and feasible policy actions to increase physical activity globally. WHO published ACTIVE a technical package to assist countries in planning and delivery of their responses. New WHO guidelines on physical activity, sedentary behavior and sleep in children under five years of age were launched in 2019.

The World Health Assembly welcomed the report of the Commission on Ending Childhood Obesity (2016) and its 6 recommendations to address the obesogenic environment and critical periods in the life course to tackle childhood obesity. The implementation plan to guide countries in taking action to implement the recommendations of the Commission was welcomed by the World Health Assembly in 2017.

April 2020

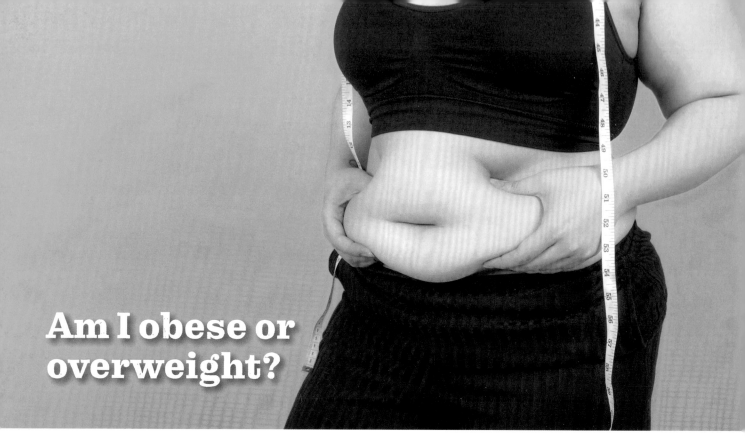

Am I obese or overweight?

This may be a strange question but do many of us really know the answer? What is classed as obesity, or am I just overweight, and is there a difference?

By Justine Clarabut

The term 'obese' describes someone that is carrying excess body fat. Obesity is usually measured using a BMI (body mass index) calculation. The guide below shows the range of BMI scores which indicate whether you are a healthy weight, overweight or obese. BMI is a universally recognised method of working out if someone is a healthy weight for their height. It is calculated by dividing your weight in kilograms by the square of your height in metres. Weight (kg) ÷ Height (m) x Height (m) = BMI (For example: 75kg ÷ 1.8m x 1.8m = 23.1)

Muscle Mass versus BMI

It is worth noting that BMI is merely an indication to see if someone is a healthy weight, it is not used to diagnose obesity! The reason being that some people are considered to be overweight according to their BMI despite having low body fat as they exhibit high levels of muscle mass! Also, as people age, they lose muscle mass, so even if they fall into the 'healthy weight range', they maybe carrying excess fat. In these situations, a BMI score is a starting point rather than a specific target and is a guide that you can discuss with your GP.

Additional ways to measure obesity

Body Fat Content (BFC) is an estimate of what proportion of the body consists of adipose (fatty tissue) as opposed to muscle, bone and other lean tissue. The readings of BFC do vary throughout the day and are dependent on the amount of water in the body.

Typical BMI scores for most adults are as follows:

18.5 to 24.9 = healthy weight

25 to 29.9 = overweight

30 to 39.9 = obese

40 or above = severely obese

Hip to waist ratio is another measurement that indicates whether someone is obese. Waist measurement divided by hip measurement. For example, a person with a 30' (76 cm) waist and 38' (97 cm) hips has a waist-hip ratio of about 0.78. A healthy waist to hip ratio for women is under .85 and for men is .90 or less

According to the NHS, men whose waist size is 94 cm or more and women whose waist size of 80 cm or more, are at a higher risk of developing obesity-related health problems.

Visceral and subcutaneous fat

Not all fat is visible. Fat can be stored in the abdominal cavity surrounding internal organs such as liver, pancreas and intestines. Visceral fat can affect how our hormones function and is sometimes referred to as 'active fat'. This is associated with a greater risk of metabolic and cardiovascular diseases. Subcutaneous fat is stored just under the skin and is the type of fat that we may be able to feel on our limbs. There is a difference between visceral fat and subcutaneous fat. A stomach that is growing can be the result of both types of fat.

The risks of being obese or overweight

Being overweight or obese increases the risk of heart disease, stroke, type II diabetes, high blood pressure (hypertension), kidney disease and some types of cancer. Carrying excess weight can also put pressure on joints, cause breathlessness and affect mobility!

Obesity can also affect our mental health causing depression, low self esteem and psychological problems. There is also the question of which came first – poor mental health which caused excess weight gain or vice versa! Each condition continually aggravates the other creating a vicious cycle.

Causes of obesity

Very simply, consuming foods that are high in calories (energy in) and then not burning off that energy through exercise and movement (energy out), will cause the body to store fat.

However, there are factors other than just poor diet, lack of exercise and inactivity. Genetic traits, and certain illnesses, can also increase the risk of obesity making it harder to maintain a healthy weight.

References:

https://www.nhs.uk/conditions/obesity/

https://fitnessgenes.com/blog/sex-hormones-visceral-fat-and-insulin/

3 January 2020

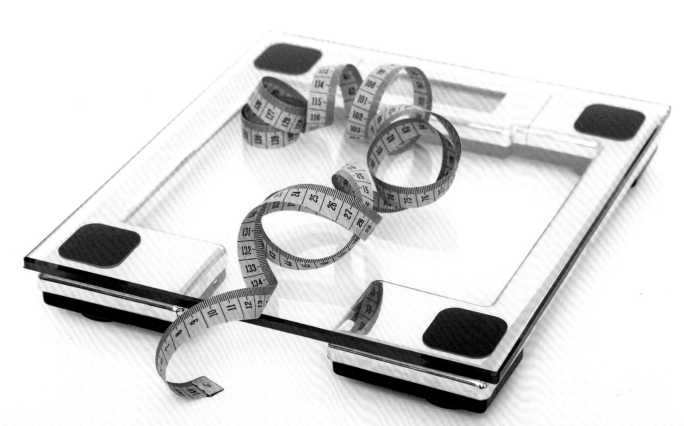

Statistics on obesity

An extract from *Statistics on Obesity, Physical Activity and Diet, England, 2020.*

Key Facts

11,117 hospital admissions directly attributable to obesity

An increase of 4% on 2017/18, when there were 10,660 admissions

876 thousand hospital admissions where obesity was a factor

An increase of 23% on 2017/18, when there were 711 thousand admissions

The majority of adults were overweight or obese; 67% of men and 60% of women.

This included 26% of men and 29% of women who were obese.

20% of year 6 children were classified as obese

Prevalence was over twice as high in the most deprived areas than the least deprived areas.

67% of adults were considered active (as per government guidelines)

47% of children and young people were meeting the current physical activity guidelines.

Adult overweight and obesity

Overweight and obesity are terms that refer to an excess of body fat and they usually relate to increased weight-for-height. The most common method of measuring obesity is the Body Mass Index (BMI).

BMI = Person's weight (kg) / Person's height (in metres)².

In adults, a BMI of 25kg/m² to 29.9kg/m² means that person is considered to be overweight, a BMI of 30kg/m² or higher means that person is considered to be obese. A BMI of 40kg/m² or higher means that person is considered to be morbidly obese. The National Institute for Health and Clinical Excellence (NICE) recommends the use of BMI in conjunction with waist circumference as the method of measuring overweight and obesity and determining health risks.

BMI does not distinguish between mass due to body fat and mass due to muscular physique, nor the distribution of fat. In order to measure abdominal obesity, waist circumference is measured, and categorised into desirable, high and very high, by sex-specific thresholds (cm):

♦ Men: Desirable = Less than 94, High = 94-102, Very high = More than 102

♦ Women: Desirable = Less than 80, High = 80-88, Very high = More than 88

The main source of the data on overweight and obesity information is the Health Survey for England (HSE), and covers adults aged 16 and over.

Overweight and obesity prevalence

Prevalence by gender

Overall, 67% of men and 60% of women were classed as overweight or obese. Being overweight but not obese was more common among men than women. However, obesity (including morbid obesity) was more common in women than men.

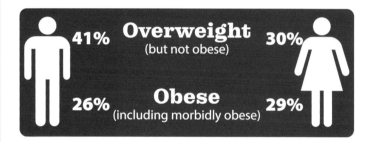

Prevalence by region (overweight or obese)

The proportion of adults who were overweight or obese according to their BMI varied by region. The lowest levels were in London, and the highest levels in the North East and the West Midlands. There was no statistically significant variation for obesity.

Prevalence by region (overweight or obese)
Regional prevalence data has been age standardised.

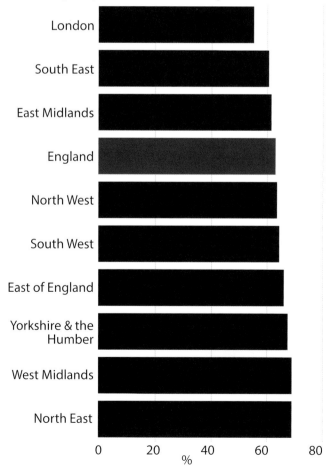

Prevalence by age

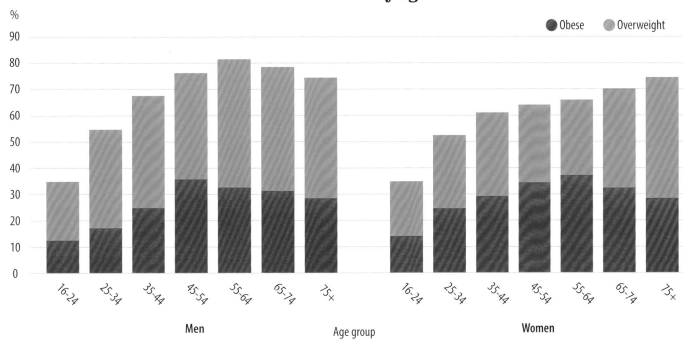

Men · Age group · Women

Prevalence by age

The proportion of adults who were overweight or obese increased with age among both men and women. It was highest among men aged between 55 and 64 (82%), and women aged between 65 and 74 (70%).

Obesity prevalence in the UK compared with other Organisation for Economic Co-operation and Development (OECD) countries

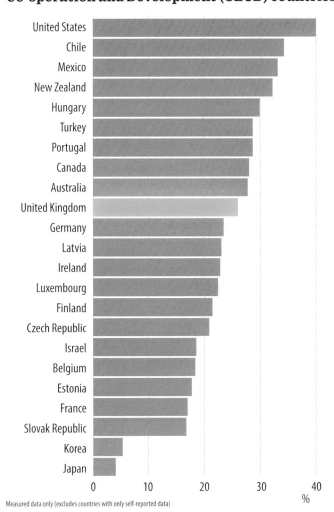

Measured data only (excludes countries with only self-reported data)

The proportion of adults who were obese also increased with age and was highest among men aged between 45 and 54 (36%), and among women aged between 55 and 64 (37%).

The UK reports an adult obesity level of 26%. This is 14 percentage points lower than the USA which reports the highest adult obesity level.

Japan and Korea report obesity levels of less than 10%.

Childhood overweight and obesity

The main source for this part is the National Child Measurement Programme for England (NCMP) which includes nearly all children in reception year (aged 4-5) and year 6 (aged 10-11). 95% of eligible children were measured in 2018/19.

Health Survey for England (HSE) also collects data on childhood obesity, covering all children aged 2-15, although as a sample it has much lower coverage than NCMP and therefore the estimates are less precise.

NCMP and HSE collect height and weight measurements to calculate BMI for each child. BMI (adjusted for age and sex) is recommended as a practical estimate of overweight and obesity in children as it takes into account different growth patterns in boys and girls at different ages.

Each age and sex group needs its own level of classification and this section uses the British 1990 growth reference (UK90) to describe childhood overweight and obesity.

Overweight and obesity prevalence

These are some of the outcomes from the National Child Measurement Programme publication for 2018/19:

♦ For reception year, obesity prevalence was 9.7%, from 9.5% in 2017/18.

♦ For year 6, obesity prevalence was 20.2%, which was similar to 2017/18.

♦ Obesity prevalence was higher for boys than girls in both age groups.

Childhood overweight and obesity

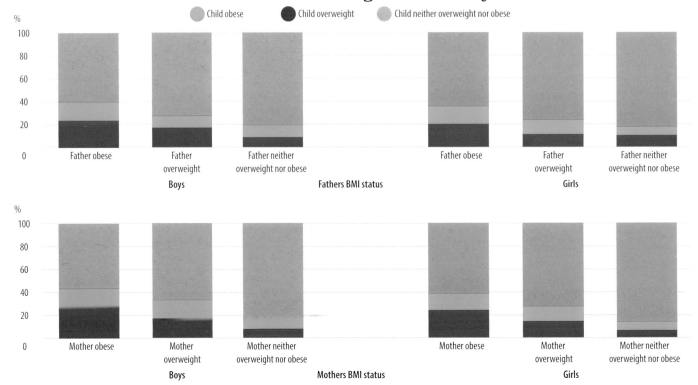

● Child obese　　● Child overweight　　● Child neither overweight nor obese

Boys — Fathers BMI status — **Girls**
(Father obese / Father overweight / Father neither overweight nor obese)

Boys — Mothers BMI status — **Girls**
(Mother obese / Mother overweight / Mother neither overweight nor obese)

♦ For children living in the most deprived areas obesity prevalence was more than double that of those living in the least deprived areas, for both reception and year 6.

Parents of overweight and obese children

Based on data from 2017 and 2018 combined, children's overweight and obesity was associated with that of their parents.

26% of children of obese mothers were also obese, compared with 16% of children whose mothers were overweight but not obese, and 7% of children whose mothers were neither overweight nor obese.

Children of obese mothers were less likely to be a healthy weight (58%) than children whose mothers were overweight but not obese (69%) or those whose mothers were neither overweight nor obese (83%).

The pattern was similar for both boys and girls.

Similarly, 22% of children of obese fathers were themselves obese, compared with 14% of children whose fathers were overweight but not obese, and 9% of children whose fathers were neither overweight nor obese.

61% of children of obese fathers were a healthy weight, compared to 74% of children whose fathers were overweight but not obese. 81% of children were a healthy weight whose fathers were neither overweight nor obese.

5 May 2020

Severe child obesity highest in Greece, Italy and Spain amid decline of Mediterranean diet, WHO report shows

Malta has highest rate of severely obese children with 5.5 per cent of six- to nine-year-olds affected, but southern Europe has higher rates than western states.

By Alex Matthews-King, Health Correspondent

Mediterranean nations whose diets have long been held up as benchmarks for healthy living have the highest rates of severe child obesity in Europe, the World Health Organisation (WHO) has warned.

A report taking in data from 21 European nations lays bare the crisis in southern states, with more than 4 per cent of primary school age children severely obese in Greece, Italy, Spain and San Marino.

With more than 5.5 per cent of children affected, Malta had the highest rates of severe obesity in the study, which is being presented at the European Congress on Obesity in Glasgow on Tuesday.

While countries in western and northern Europe, including Belgium, Ireland and Norway, had severe obesity rates below 2 per cent, some notoriously overweight states – such as the UK – were not included. France, Germany and Russia were also left out of the study.

Researchers said one factor was likely to be the 'decline' in the idealised Mediterranean diet, high in whole grains, nuts, vegetables, olive oil and fish.

Many countries are now seeing the effects of an influx of cheap, high calorie convenience foods and some, such as Denmark and the UK, have introduced taxes on high sugar or high-fat items.

Where childhood obesity is most prevalent in Europe
Share of 6 to 9 year olds considered obese in European countries (2015-2017)*

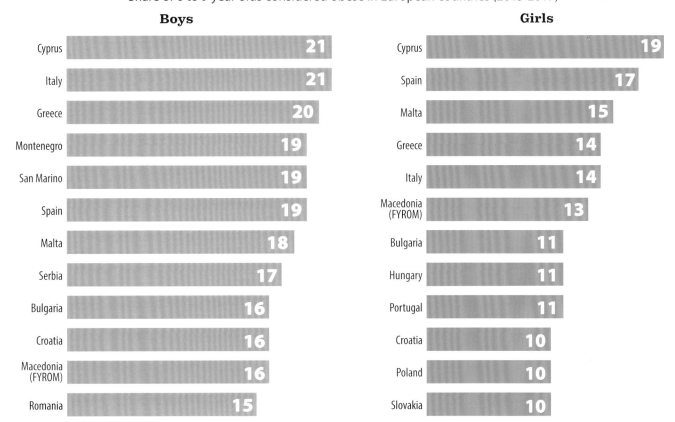

Boys

Country	%
Cyprus	21
Italy	21
Greece	20
Montenegro	19
San Marino	19
Spain	19
Malta	18
Serbia	17
Bulgaria	16
Croatia	16
Macedonia (FYROM)	16
Romania	15

Girls

Country	%
Cyprus	19
Spain	17
Malta	15
Greece	14
Italy	14
Macedonia (FYROM)	13
Bulgaria	11
Hungary	11
Portugal	11
Croatia	10
Poland	10
Slovakia	10

* Based on the 2007 WHO recommended growth reference. Age of children varies between countries, within the span of 6 to 9 years.
Not all European countries included in the research, e.g. the UK and Germany

Source: World Health Organization

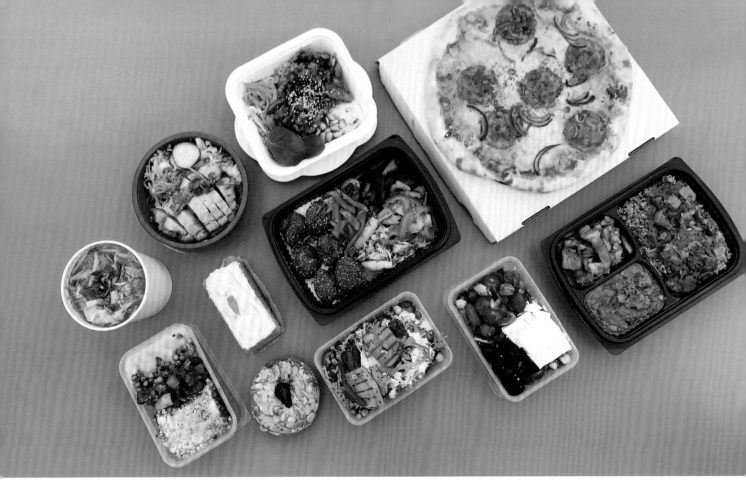

Other studies have found similarly high rates of child and adult obesity in southern Mediterranean nations.

But the research, led by Dr João Breda, head of the WHO's European office for Prevention and Control of Noncommunicable Diseases, is the first to look specifically at 'severe' child obesity. This is defined differently from adults but roughly requires them to have a body mass index higher than 19 out of 20 children in their age group.

Dr Breda and colleagues said an explanation for higher rates of obesity in southern Europe 'remains elusive', though there are several possible explanations.

'The loss of the Mediterranean diet in southern European countries could be linked to this severe obesity problem,' the authors said.

Though it could also be a result of 'lower height-for-age found in southern Europe', higher birth weights, reduced sleep duration and different patterns for meals and physical activity.

Higher rates of maternal education were another factor that reduced the risk of severe obesity, the report found.

The authors warn that without action the same pattern could develop in other nations with traditionally Mediterranean diets and habits, such as Albania and Moldova.

'Without timely, appropriate and effective policy measures to prevent obesity, there is a risk that prevalence rates in these countries will eventually match the levels seen in other European countries,' the authors said.

The study used data from 636,933 six- to nine-year-olds, and the findings indicate that there are at least 400,000 children who are already severely obese of a total 13.7 million six- to nine-year-olds in the 21 countries included in the study.

'Severe obesity is a serious public health issue and the results of this study show that a large number of children in Europe suffer from it,' the authors concluded.

'Given its impact on education, health, social care and the economy, obesity needs to be addressed via a range of approaches, from prevention to early diagnosis and treatment.'

30 April 2019

Obesity is not inevitable: a personal view

By John Newton

Obesity is not inevitable for individuals or for countries, but neither is it easy to avoid or reverse it. The environment we all live in can often make it hard for all of us to consistently make healthy choices these days.

And that is why many of us today are carrying excess weight. Almost 7 out of 10 men, and 6 out of 10 women in England are overweight or living with obesity. Too many children are now obese before they reach school age and more become obese while they are at school – this is a tragedy – and the impact of obesity is even worse in disadvantaged groups and some ethnic minorities.

Obesity matters – it affects our health, our life chances and our self-esteem. It makes the work of the NHS and care services more difficult. It is a pressure on the economy.

Living with obesity increases the risk of type 2 diabetes, many cancers, cardiovascular diseases, liver disease and respiratory diseases, and has other effects for example on joint and back pain and on mental health. Losing weight if you are living with obesity improves health – for example for people with pre-diabetes, losing one kilo reduces risk of diabetes by 16%. Weight loss of 5-10% lowers blood pressure and so reduces risk of heart disease.

Thirty years ago, it was different – something has changed – how has this happened?

Why do people become overweight and obese?

To put it simply, people become overweight because they eat and drink more calories than they need. Inactivity is important, but it is not the main problem. We mainly eat and drink what is made easily available and promoted to us in supermarkets, restaurants, pubs and takeaways.

Attractive high calorie food and drink has become much more widely available in the last three decades – over the years it has become cheaper in real terms and much more intensively advertised and promoted. That is very likely to be one of the main causes of the rise in obesity.

Coronavirus has been a shock

It has been a shock to the country that so many people have died in the UK from coronavirus – more than in other countries. We can all be affected by this new disease but people living in deprived communities and those from ethnic minorities have suffered especially badly from coronavirus.

Overweight and obesity is one factor that explains why some people suffer more than others and is something that we can change.

Risk of a positive test and outcome of COVID-19 is worse according to weight. With a BMI of 35-40 risk of death from COVID-19 is up by 40% – with a BMI over 40 it almost doubles. In intensive care units, 8% of critically ill patients with COVID-19 were morbidly obese compared with 3% of the general population.

We can do better on obesity

We need to show that the UK can do better, and we can do better than this on obesity.

We especially want to do better for our children and for people living in deprived communities in our country – this is not just about caring for our own health.

Many of us have been motivated to do something about our health by coronavirus. Downloads of PHE's physical activity app almost doubled during lockdown, but most people cannot control their weight on their own – help is needed.

Government has a central role to act to make the healthier choice the easier choice. That means substantially changing the way food and drink are advertised, promoted and sold across the board. Many of the policies that matter and will make an impact lie outside the health sector, so promoting a healthy weight is a whole of government issue.

We have a good track record in other areas of public health. Other countries envy what the UK has achieved on tobacco control and on salt reduction – it has required sustained policy effort in those areas over many years and we can do the same on obesity. It will not be easy, but it will be well worth it.

There is synergy with other policy drivers – safeguarding the environment and net zero carbon for example. Increasing physical activity also has other benefits.

The NHS can help significantly as a brand leader and by providing services, local government commissions health checks, and employers and civil society also need to play their part.

Weight management services and other individual level interventions are needed and do help those who receive them, but we need to do this together with other measures to change the underlying causes of the trend in overweight and obesity and to support people in maintaining a healthier weight.

Sum up

Coronavirus has been a shock in part because this country has suffered badly compared with many others. The UK needs to respond to improve health and obesity is an area where we can do much better.

Cross-government policy action can significantly help improve the way we eat and drink as a nation. Nothing else will make as much difference to ensuring a healthy weight.

That is why now is the right time to focus the nation's mind on how they can reach and maintain a healthy weight with the government supporting them in their weight loss, alongside introducing policies to make the healthier choice the easier choice. The public are likely to respond well now to a publicity campaign to raise the profile of obesity both in relation to COVID-19 and to general health.

25 July 2020

Free school meals: the lifelong impact of childhood food poverty

An article from The Conversation.

THE CONVERSATION

By Regina Keith, Senior Lecturer in Food, Nutrition and Public Health, University of Westminster

The coronavirus pandemic has had a devastating impact on household food security in the UK. Five million families have encountered food insecurity, and 200,000 children are missing meals every day.

Despite a campaign led by Manchester United and England footballer Marcus Rashford, the UK government has voted against extending free school meals to children during the autumn half-term holiday and future holidays until Easter 2021. Rashford is now leading a concerted effort from councils, charities and businesses to provide free meals over the school holiday.

'Holiday hunger' – when children go without the food normally provided to families during school term time – is an increasingly recognised issue. If children are not given the nutrition they need, there are long-term effects on their health.

Mind and body

In the short term, children who are living in food-insecure families are more likely to suffer from education losses.

Research from the US showed that after the summer holidays, children had lost an average of one month's worth of skills learned at school, and that poorer children may fare worst.

When children do not have enough to eat, they are less likely to achieve their developmental goals on time, or to achieve their potential at school.

Children experiencing food insecurity are more likely to suffer from anxiety and stress, and hunger in childhood has been linked to depression and suicidal episodes in teenagers. Hunger is also linked to increased levels of chronic illnesses such as asthma.

Children require essential nutrients from food, such as zinc, iron, selenium, protein and iodine, to support their brain growth. The supply of these nutrients affects the functioning adult the child will become.

Another vital nutrient is vitamin D, found in foods such as oily fish, red meat and egg yolks. Vitamin D is essential

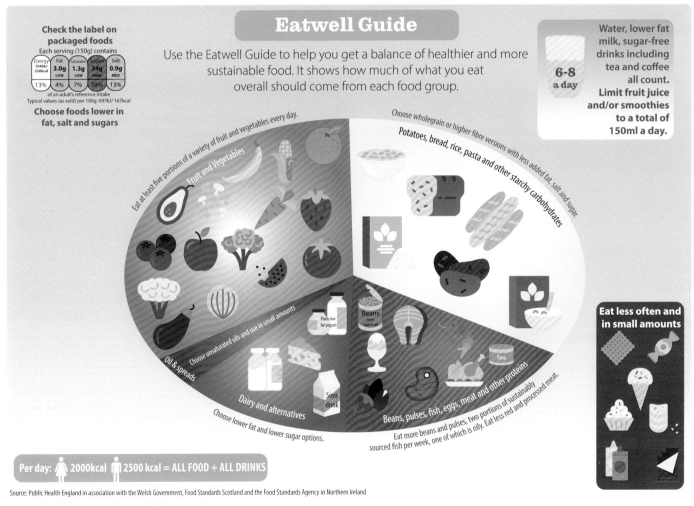

Check the label on packaged foods

Each serving (150g) contains

Energy 1046kJ 250kcal	Fat 3.0g LOW	Saturates 1.3g LOW	Sugars 34g HIGH	Salt 0.9g MED
	13%	4%	7%	38%	13%

of an adult's reference intake
Typical values (as sold) per 100g: 697kJ/ 167kcal

Choose foods lower in fat, salt and sugars

Eatwell Guide

Use the Eatwell Guide to help you get a balance of healthier and more sustainable food. It shows how much of what you eat overall should come from each food group.

Water, lower fat milk, sugar-free drinks including tea and coffee all count. Limit fruit juice and/or smoothies to a total of 150ml a day.

6-8 a day

Eat at least five portions of a variety of fruit and vegetables every day.

Fruit and Vegetables

Choose wholegrain or higher fibre versions with less added fat, salt and sugar

Potatoes, bread, rice, pasta and other starchy carbohydrates

Choose unsaturated oils and use in small amounts

Oil & spreads

Plain low fat yogurt

Beans lower in salt

Soya drink

Dairy and alternatives

Choose lower fat and lower sugar options.

Tuna

Beans, pulses, fish, eggs, meat and other proteins

Eat more beans and pulses, two portions of sustainably sourced fish per week, one of which is oily. Eat less red and processed meat.

Eat less often and in small amounts

Per day: 2000kcal 2500 kcal = ALL FOOD + ALL DRINKS

Source: Public Health England in association with the Welsh Government, Food Standards Scotland and the Food Standards Agency in Northern Ireland

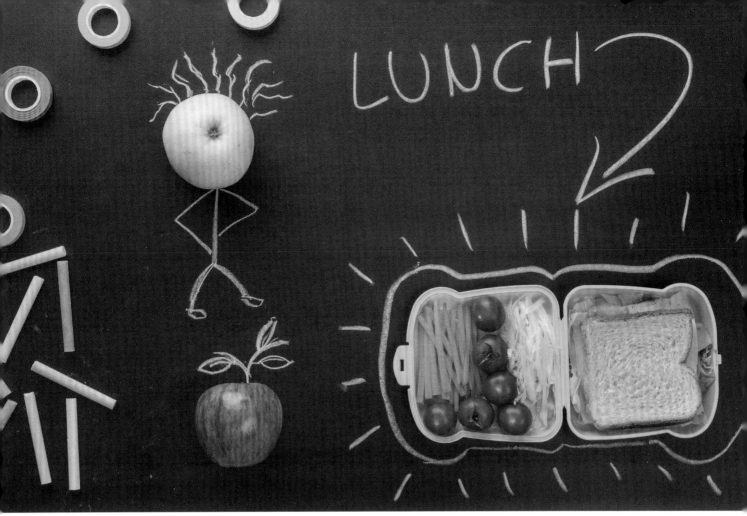

for bone growth in children, and it is linked to enhanced protection against illnesses by reducing inflammation and promoting immune function. Research has also shown that vitamin D may protect against respiratory illnesses. In the UK, it has been estimated that 16% of children do not have enough vitamin D.

Poor nutrition has an impact across generations. Mothers who are lacking in iron are more likely to have children who do not grow well during pregnancy and are born with low birth weight. These infants often have developmental problems and are more likely to suffer from infectious diseases and death in childhood.

Mothers who were undernourished as children are also more likely to have underweight babies. The long-term impacts of low birth weight are stark, and include increased rates of high blood pressure, diabetes, coronary artery disease and obesity. Research has also found a link between low birth weight and heart disease in adults.

Five a day

The government advises that children need to eat a balanced diet. This is set out in the Eatwell guidelines developed by Public Health England. The guidelines suggest eating at least five portions of fruit and vegetables a day. Fruit and veg contain essential nutrients such as zinc and iron, which help the body grow and fight diseases.

For many families, though, meeting this target is not easy. In fact, a quarter of secondary school children in the UK eat less than one portion of fruit or vegetables a day.

In 2018, the Food Foundation charity published a report showing that following the Eatwell guide was likely to be unaffordable for families living on a low income. The report calculated that families earning less than £15,860 would need to spend 42% of their income (after housing) on food to meet the Eatwell guidelines.

The evidence is clear: children not eating a healthy diet will not perform as well at school as those who are well nourished. They are more likely to suffer from mental health problems such as stress, and as they age they will be more likely to suffer from diseases such as cancer, diabetes, heart disease and obesity.

The coronavirus pandemic has left many parents struggling to feed their children. The UK is faced with the challenge of how to protect its most vulnerable population.

23 October 2020

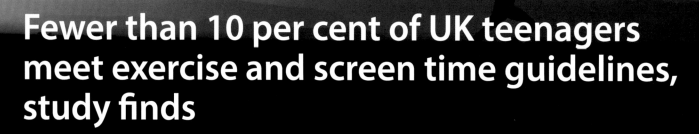

Fewer than 10 per cent of UK teenagers meet exercise and screen time guidelines, study finds

British teenagers spend too long looking at screens and not enough time exercising or sleeping.

By Alex Shipman

British teenagers spend too long looking at screens and not enough time exercising or sleeping – with less than ten per cent meeting the recommended guidelines.

Research found children aged between five and 17 should spend an hour a day doing moderate to vigorous exercise and no more than two hours a day in front of a screen.

It tracks participants' movements over 24 hours – and recommends they sleep for at least eight hours a night.

But only 9.7 per cent of 14-year-olds in the UK manage all three recommendations, a new study published in the journal Jama Pediatrics suggests.

More than three-quarters of teenagers spend more than two hours a day interacting with screens, it adds.

The latest study is based on data collected between January 2015 and March 2016 from 14-year-olds in the UK, *The Guardian* reports.

The authors noted: 'Screen time was the main driver of not meeting all three recommendations.'

Participants reported their average daily screen time – including TV, tablet and computer use – alongside bedtime and waking times on an average school night.

Their levels of exercise were also monitored through an activity tracker worn on both a weekday and a weekend day.

Other data was gathered through questionnaires and measurements, with almost 4,000 teens analysed in total.

The results reveal almost 90% reported sleeping for more than eight hours on a school night, but only 23% said they spent two hours or less a day interacting with screens.

Activity tracker data revealed that 41% of teenagers met the recommended level of moderate to vigorous physical activity.

Only 9.7% of participants met recommendations for all three behaviours.

The team found that teenagers with symptoms of depression were less likely to meet all three recommendations.

Overweight girls and obese boys were also less likely to meet all three.

26 August 2019

Four in five teenagers not doing enough exercise, says World Health Organization

Girls found to lag behind boys in staying active.

By Samuel Osborne

Four out of five teenagers in the UK are not doing enough exercise, according to a report from the World Health Organisation (WHO).

Girls were found to lag behind boys in staying active, a trend one of the researchers described as 'concerning'.

The figures are the first global estimates on physical activity among 11 to 17-year-olds, involving 1.6 million students from 146 countries.

Worldwide, girls on average were found to be less active than boys, with 84.7 per cent failing to reach the recommended exercise targets, which is slightly lower than the UK figure of 85.4 per cent.

Dr Leanne Riley, a researcher at the WHO and one of the study authors, said: 'The trend of girls being less active than boys is concerning.

'More opportunities to meet the needs and interests of girls are needed to attract and sustain their participation in physical activity through adolescence and into adulthood.'

The WHO recommends adolescents take part in an hour of moderate-to-vigorous physical activity – which can include walking, cycling or playing games – each day.

The new analysis, published in Lancet Adolescent And Child Health, found that 81 per cent of students around the world are not meeting these requirements.

Boys in the Philippines (93 per cent) and girls in South Korea (97 per cent) were found to be the most inactive in the study. Although Bangladesh had the lowest levels of inactivity for boys and girls, figures showed two in three children (66 per cent) were not doing an hour a day of exercise.

The authors said levels of insufficient physical activity in adolescents continued to be extremely high, raising concerns about their current and future health.

Dr Regina Guthold, a WHO researcher and one of the study authors, said: 'Urgent policy action to increase physical activity is needed now, particularly to promote and retain girls' participation in physical activity.'

Writing in a linked comment in the journal, Dr Mark Tremblay, of the Children's Hospital of Eastern Ontario Research Institute in Canada, said physical inactivity is the fourth leading risk factor for premature death worldwide.

He said: 'The electronic revolution has fundamentally transformed people's movement patterns by changing where and how they live, learn, work, play and travel, progressively isolating them indoors.

'People sleep less, sit more, walk less frequently, drive more regularly and do less physical activity than they used to.'

22 November 2019

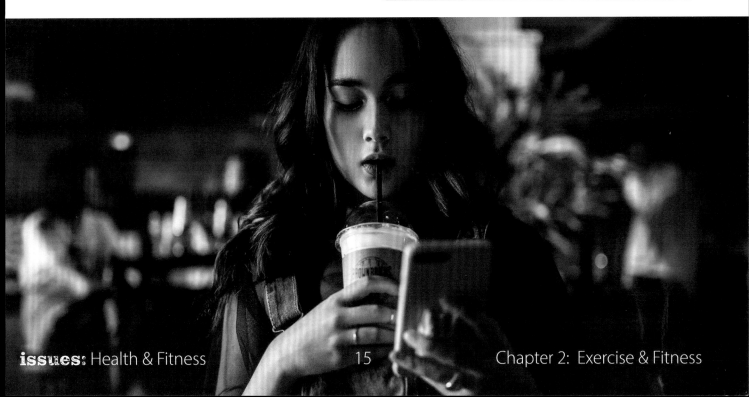

Physical activity

An extract from *Statistics on Obesity, Physical Activity and Diet, England, 2020.*

The health benefits of a physically active lifestyle are well documented and there is a large amount of evidence to suggest that regular activity is related to reduced incidence of many chronic conditions. Physical activity contributes to a wide range of health benefits and regular physical activity can improve health outcomes irrespective of whether individuals achieve weight loss.

In 2019 new guidelines on the amount of activity recommended for health were published by the Chief Medical Officers of the four UK countries. This states that:

♦ Adults (aged 19 and over) should aim to be active daily. Over a week, activity should add up to at least 150 minutes of moderate intensity activity or 75 minutes of vigorous intensity activity per week, or a combination of both.

♦ Adults should also aim to build strength on at least two days a week.

♦ Children and young people (aged 5 to 18) should aim to be physically active for at least 60 minutes per day across the week.

Adult physical activity

Adult physical activity by gender

In the 12 months to November 2019, around two thirds of adults (67%) were considered active as per the government guidelines. 21% were considered to be inactive (<30 minutes on average per week).

Adult physical activity by gender

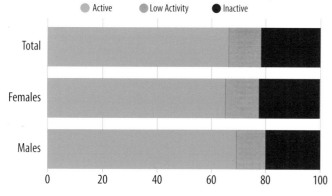

Men (70%) were more likely to be active than women (65%).

Adult physical activity by age group

The most active group are those aged 19-24 with 74% considered active. After this levels remain similar (between 68% and 71%), until a decline at ages 75-84 (53% active) and age 85+ (31% active).

Adult physical activity by deprivation level

Deprivation level is based on Index of Multiple Deprivation scores for English Lower Super Output Areas, grouped into deciles.

Activity levels decrease as deprivation increases, from 73% active in the least deprived areas, to 57% in the most deprived areas.

Adult physical activity by age group

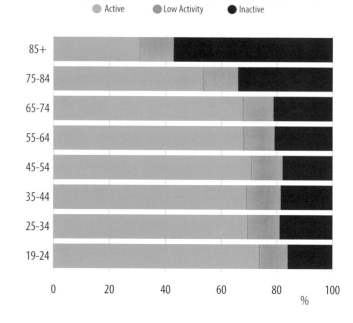

Adult physical activity by deprivation level

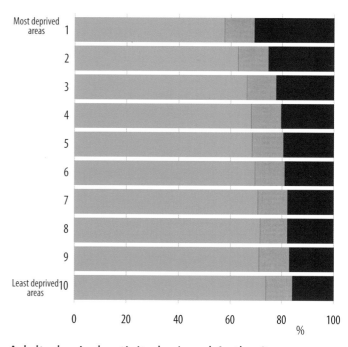

Adult physical activity by Local Authority

The proportion of adults classified as active ranged from 47% to 82% across Local Authorities.

City of London, Wandsworth, Richmond upon Thames. Brighton & Hove, Bath & North East Somerset, Islington, Wokingham, and York all had proportions active above 75%.

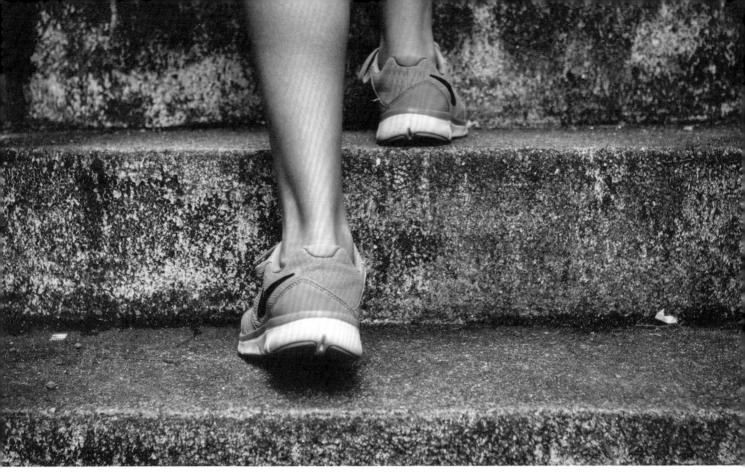

Childhood physical activity by gender

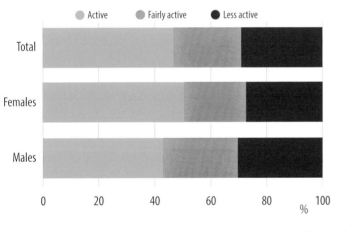

Legend: Active · Fairly active · Less active

Categories (top to bottom): Total, Females, Males
X-axis: 0 20 40 60 80 100 %

Childhood physical activity by family affluence

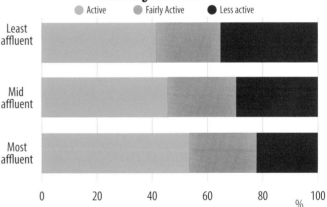

Legend: Active · Fairly Active · Less active

Categories (top to bottom): Least affluent, Mid affluent, Most affluent
X-axis: 0 20 40 60 80 100 %

Barking & Dagenham, Stoke-on-Trent, Sandwell, and Rotherham had proportions active of less than 55%.

Childhood physical activity

Childhood physical activity by gender

Based on the 2018/19 academic year, 47% of children and young people are meeting the current guidelines of taking part in sport and physical activity for an average of 60 minutes or more every day. This is an increase from 43% in 2017/18.

A further 24% are fairly active, taking part for an average of between 30-59 minutes per day, whilst 29% do less than an average of 30 minutes a day.

Boys (51%) are more likely to be active than girls (43%).

Childhood physical activity by family affluence

The Family Affluence Scale provides an indication of the social status of children and young people's families. The scale is derived from a series of questions about their home and family such as car ownership, computers, and foreign holidays.

Results show some significant inequalities in activity levels, based on family income.

In total, 35% of children in the least affluent families do fewer than 30 minutes of activity a day, compared to 22% of children from the most affluent families.

5 May 2020

Physical activity
for children & young people (5-18 years)

Builds confidence & social skills

Develops co-ordination

Improves concentration & learning

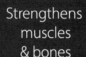

Strengthens muscles & bones

Improves health & fitness

  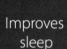

Maintains healthy weight

Improves sleep

Makes you feel good

Be physically active

Spread activity throughout the day

All activities should make you breathe faster and feel warmer

Aim for an average of at least **60** minutes per day across the week

Play

Run/walk

Bike

Active travel

Swim

Skate

Activities to develop movement skills, and muscle and bone strength **across week**

Sport

PE

Skip

Climb

Reduce inactivity

Workout

Dance

Get strong

Move more

The above information is reprinted with kind permission from Gov UK.
© Crown copyright 2021
This information is licensed under the Open Government Licence v3.0
To view this licence, visit http://www.nationalarchives.gov.uk/doc/open-government-licence/ **OGL**

Source: UK Chief Medical Officers' Physical Activity Guidelines, 2019

www.gov.uk

Why exercise is important, but nutrition is even better: sure-fire ways to help our health

By Daniel Hunt, Freelance Consultant in Public Health Policy

As the COVID-19 pandemic has starkly reminded us, the basic functioning of the economy and the building blocks of a fair society depend on good health. Many people have been put at greater risk of the virus because of underlying health conditions that could have been prevented, many of them linked to overweight and obesity.

And meanwhile, shockingly high rates of children's obesity continue to persist, even among those as young as primary school age. In this blog, we reflect on what we know about how exercise and nutrition affect our ability to keep a healthy weight, particularly among children, and consider some ways the government can act.

Fit as a fiddle: the many benefits of exercise

Keeping physically active is vital to help us prevent lots of different diseases. For all of us, this includes cardiovascular disease, type 2 diabetes, some cancers, and osteoporosis, as well as improving glucose homeostasis and bone density. Exercise is associated with a 'better general and health-related quality of life' for those with mental health conditions, while there is also a small but consistent evidence base that keeping fit can help reduce weight gain for women in pregnancy.

And there's plenty of benefits for children. Moderate or vigorous exercise can strengthen children's cardiovascular and respiratory systems, as well as their bone health. Exercise is also positively linked with improved mental health outcomes and education attainment. And happily, even small amounts of exercise are better than none.

We also know that far too many children are not getting as much physical activity as they should – a problem likely to have been compounded during COVID-19 lockdown. And far too many children – more than four in five in England – fail to meet the recommended amount of physical activity. These numbers get worse with increasing rates of deprivation, condemning the poorest children to worse life-chances.

However, while Public Health England recognise that our activity levels are around 20% lower than in the 1960s, they have remained relatively stable over the last decade. In short, while there's clearly so much more room for exercise, there's not clear evidence that children's recent exercise levels are decreasing.

Given around one-third of kids have a weight classed as overweight or obese before they even leave primary school, this suggests that there's something else at play. It's not just exercise: a systematic review looking at multiple studies investigating the link between how much a child exercises and their weight, found 'physical activity is not strongly prospectively related with [child weight]'.

Full of beans: good nutrition is even better

Unfortunately, exercise isn't the silver bullet for reducing obesity. To understand what has the most effect on rising rates of obesity, the UK Government's Behavioural Insights Team looked at the possible factors. Their conclusion on if a lack of exercise was driving obesity was clear: 'we do not consider this to be a plausible argument'.

For all UK nations, research shows what we eat, rather than a lack of exercise, causes significantly more impact on our health. Across the population of England in 2016, 5.5 times more years of life were lost from diseases linked to what we eat, rather than low levels of physical activity. And in Northern Ireland, Scotland and Wales, this was even higher, at 6.3 times, 6.5 times and 8.1 times respectively.

These findings match the global picture. The most recent Global Burden of Disease study, an analysis of the health of 195 countries, found that poor diet creates the biggest cluster of risk factors for health of any behavioural, environmental, occupational or metabolic risk. And a similar global study of 69 countries looking at what was responsible for driving obesity around the world, found increases in the food supply were more impactful than a lack of exercise, 'especially [so] in high-income countries' like the UK.

Essentially, the reason obesity and diet-related diseases are driven by what we eat, rather than how much we exercise, is what's called 'caloric overconsumption'. In their report looking at the drivers of obesity, the Behavioural Insights Team estimated as a population, we consume 30% to 50% more calories than are reported in official statistics. To put it

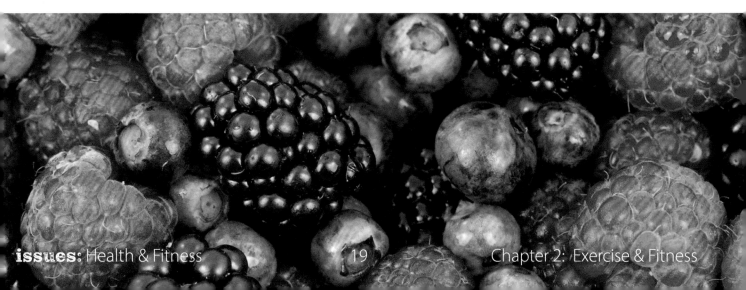

another way, if we actually consumed as few calories as we say we do, we would be losing weight across the UK, rather than gaining it.

One reason for this is likely to be how we perceive the amount of energy we burn when exercising. Typically, we overestimate the calories we burn through exercise – in part because tools like fitness trackers are good for measuring heart rate, but have been found to overestimate calories burned through physical activity. As a consequence, this might lead to us eating more overall after exercise.

Another key problem here is how foods are made and labelled. Some food corporations take a dishonest approach to their products, either by packing them full of hidden saturated fat, sugar and salt, or not following the established best-practice of having clear traffic-light labelling. This can be deceiving – making us think products are healthier than they are, and disguising calories from the consumer.

More broadly, these companies take every opportunity to market and promote their products. And for them, exercise is fair game. We will return to this point in the second part of this blog.

To tackle children's obesity, exercise is good, but nutrition is even better

Children have a right to grow up in a society that looks after them. They cannot decide what we consider acceptable as a society. They don't get to choose how many junk food ads they see. In short, they have no control over the commercial forces trying to recruit them as customers of tomorrow.

Because we're talking about protecting child health, there's no point wasting time on ineffective interventions. What's more, it's dangerous to do so. A decade of inaction from the food industry, through voluntary targets and public pledges, have not delivered a meaningful change in their corporate conduct. At the same time, children have needlessly been exposed to diseases that could affect the rest of their lives.

Industry's inability to deliver progress sits in sharp contrast to the effectiveness of the leadership of the UK Government, and the benefits already being felt from the Soft Drinks Industry Levy.

What's more, we're ready to go. The Government has already consulted on a range of evidence-based measures to protect children and make it easier for us to eat healthily, and promote the idea that food is meant to nourish and sustain us, not make us sick. These consultations are eagerly awaited, and long overdue.

In recent weeks there have been signs that the Government is ready to consider comprehensive action to address obesity. Exercise has an important role in good health, and encouraging it is very important. But ultimately, if we're to make the meaningful changes that help us reach a healthy weight, it's crystal clear that the food environment needs an overhaul.

10 June 2020

9 proven benefits of physical activity

Physical activity refers to all the movement we carry out throughout the day, such as doing housework, bringing in shopping, walking to work and doing exercise like playing a sport or going to the gym. Evidence continues to mount that being physically active can benefit both body and mind, as well as reducing the risk of many diseases. Here are nine proven benefits of regular physical activity.

1. Helps maintain a healthy body weight

Low physical activity can increase someone's risk of becoming overweight or obese. While exercising alone does not necessarily lead to weight loss, in combination with a balanced calorie-controlled diet, it can support successful weight reduction. In addition, there is evidence that regular physical activity can help maintain a healthy body weight over time.

2. Lowers blood pressure

High blood pressure (or hypertension) is a risk factor for many diseases, particularly stroke and heart disease. Regular physical activity can increase your heart's strength, which reduces the effort needed to pump blood around the body. This decreases the force on your arteries, reducing blood pressure. There is good evidence that regular physical activity helps maintain a healthy blood pressure.

3. Decreases the risk of heart disease

Regular exercise, especially aerobic exercise, such as brisk walking, running and cycling, has been shown to reduce the risk of developing heart disease. This benefit is observed for people of all body sizes. People with overweight or obesity who are physically active are far less likely to get heart disease compared to those who aren't.

4. Lowers the risk of type 2 diabetes

Exercise is known to help in the regulation of blood sugar levels and improves our bodies, sensitivity to insulin. Physical inactivity, on the other hand, has been consistently shown to increase the risk of developing type 2 diabetes. Furthermore, regular exercise is often recommended to people with diabetes to aid in their control of blood sugar levels.

5. Reduces the risk of certain cancers

Cancer is a complex disease influenced by many controllable (e.g. smoking, unhealthy diet, high alcohol consumption) and uncontrollable (e.g. genetics, radiation, environmental pollutants) factors. Evidence suggests that regular moderate to vigorous exercise can help reduce our risk of developing certain types of cancers, including colon, colorectal, lung and breast cancers.

6. Increases muscle strength and function

Skeletal muscle serves many functions, it helps maintain

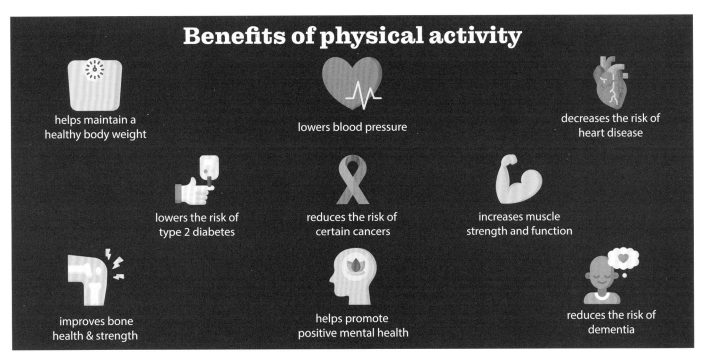

Benefits of physical activity

helps maintain a healthy body weight

lowers blood pressure

decreases the risk of heart disease

lowers the risk of type 2 diabetes

reduces the risk of certain cancers

increases muscle strength and function

improves bone health & strength

helps promote positive mental health

reduces the risk of dementia

Physical activity

moderate

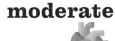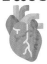

noticeably acclerates the heart rate

vs.

vigorous

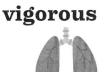

causes rapid breathing and a substantial increase in heart rate

e.g.
brisk walking, dancing, gardening, housework & domestic chores

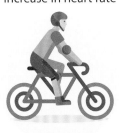

e.g.
running, fast swimming, fast cycling, competitive sports (e.g. football)

the intensity of different forms of physical activity varies between people

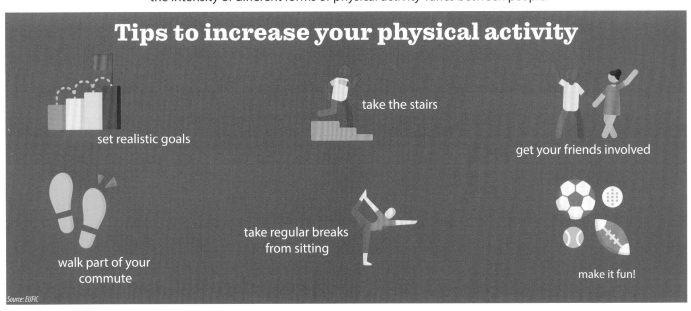

Tips to increase your physical activity

set realistic goals

take the stairs

get your friends involved

walk part of your commute

take regular breaks from sitting

make it fun!

Source: EUFIC

posture, controls movement and generates body heat. As we age, our muscle mass tends to decrease, often due to a more sedentary lifestyle. This loss of muscle mass can reduce our mobility and increase our risk of falls and muscular diseases such as sarcopenia. Regular exercise, particularly resistance training (such as lifting weights or bodyweight exercises such as squats and push-ups) can help improve muscle strength and resilience and reduce our risk of muscular disorders like sarcopenia.

7. Improves bone health and strength

Weight-bearing exercise (e.g. running, dancing), as well as resistance training, have been shown to improve bone density in adolescents and help maintain bone density in adulthood, reducing the risk of osteoporosis. This is particularly important for older adults and menopausal women as it can help to slow the natural loss of bone density that occurs with age.

8. Helps to promote positive mental health

Regular exercise has been shown to have a positive effect on our mental health and psychological well-being. The exact mechanism for which exercise benefits our mental health is not fully understood. What is known is regular exercise can promote the release of endorphins as well as help relieve stress and promote a healthy sleep pattern, which can all work together to improve our mood. In addition, there is some evidence to suggest that exercise may even help in the treatment of depression and other mental disorders.

9. Reduces the risk of dementia

Regular exercise has been consistently shown to protect against cognitive decline. Although it is still not fully understood how exercise reduces cognitive decline, recent evidence suggests that the release of proteins known as neurotrophic factors likely play an important role. These beneficial factors help promote neuron growth and repair which help support normal cognitive functioning. This may partly explain why older adults who remain physically active throughout life have a much lower risk of developing cognitive disorders such as dementia and Alzheimer's disease.

How much physical activity should we do?

The World Health Organization recommends:

We do a minimum of at least 150 minutes of moderate-intensity aerobic physical activity throughout the week or at least 75 minutes of vigorous-intensity aerobic physical activity throughout the week or an equivalent combination of moderate- and vigorous-intensity activity.

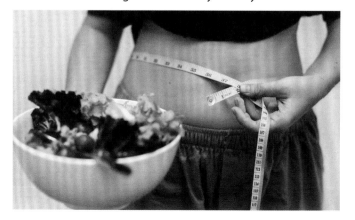

Aerobic activities should be performed in bouts of at least ten minutes' duration.

For additional health benefits, adults should aim to increase their moderate-intensity aerobic physical activity to 300 minutes per week, or 150 minutes of vigorous-intensity aerobic physical activity per week, or an equivalent combination of both moderate- and vigorous-intensity activity.

Muscle-strengthening or anaerobic activities should be done involving major muscle groups (legs, hips, back, abdomen, chest, shoulders and arms) on two or more days a week.

For people with prior health conditions, it is advised they consult a health professional before undertaking additional exercise.

Tips to increase your physical activity

In today's busy society, regular physical activity can be hard to maintain and requires both time and effort. Here are some tips to help you increase your physical activity levels:

Set realistic goals: making a commitment to increase your physical activity is an important first step. Setting a goal (e.g. get 10,000 steps every day) and planning what you need to do to achieve this goal (e.g. plan to walk part of your commute) can help keep you focused and committed.

Take the stairs: An easy way to increase your daily physical activity is to take the stairs instead of lifts or elevators wherever possible.

Get your friends involved: Exercise is better with friends, try joining a sports team or going for a run or brisk walk with a friend.

Walk part of your commute: Try getting off a stop early or parking further away and walking part of your commute.

Take regular breaks from sitting: Many of us spend most of our days seated, be it at work or at home. Try to take regular breaks to walk around and stretch your legs and avoid sitting for long periods.

Make it fun: Exercise shouldn't be a chore, much like eating a healthy balanced diet, if we don't enjoy it we won't be able to keep it up for long. Try to find an activity that you enjoy and can stick to long-term.

In summary

It seems clear that physical activity has several health benefits. However, we must not forget that it is just one part of a healthy lifestyle and for good health, we should also focus on eating a balanced diet that is rich in fruits and vegetables, whole grains, some dairy, nuts, pulses, eggs, lean meat and oily fish, and limit our intake of saturated fat, sugars and salt.

12 February 2020

5 ways exercise impacts your sleep (good and bad)

Exercise can benefit your sleep in many ways, but knowing what to do and when to do it is key to reaping the greatest rewards.

Medically reviewed by Dr Juliet McGrattan (MBChB) and words by Laura Williams

Two components of a healthy lifestyle are undoubtedly sleep and exercise, but not much is known about how they impact each other. Sleep can help performance and provides you with more energy for exercise, while a sufficient exercise routine contributes to healthy sleep patterns. But what time should we exercise for it to benefit our sleep? And can physical activity ever impede a good night's kip?

Personal trainer Laura Williams explains how to juggle your exercise routine with adequate sleep so you can make the most of your health:

1. Cardio is key for sleep quality

Research undertaken by the National Institute on Ageing found that participants who engaged in aerobic exercise (walking, treadmill, bike) up to four times a week at 75 per cent of their MHR (Maximum Heart Rate) reported better sleep quality, less daytime sleepiness and a greater sense of vitality during the day. The study also found that aerobic exercise improved the time it took to fall asleep by 14 per cent.

Cardio caution

Intensity counts when it comes to making your aerobic exercise work for your bedtime routine. Shift the tougher puff stuff to earlier in the day (see below) if you're looking to maximise results on your sleep pattern. A brisk post-dinner walk however should be just fine and add plenty of sleep-inducing bang minus the sleep-disruption buck.

2. It's all about the timing

Exercising late at night can interrupt your sleep in several different ways. Higher intensity exercise that significantly raises the heart rate not only stimulates your muscles and cardiovascular system, it also raises your body temperature which should remain lower close to bedtime. You may also find that the adrenaline produced from a higher intensity workout makes it more difficult to unwind too.

Timing tip

If you find your sleep suffers after an evening workout, try shifting your exercise session to earlier in the day. Not possible? Time to tick the temperature and nutrition boxes. A post-exercise shower should help to reduce body temperature while ensuring you head to bed neither stuffed from your post-workout snack, nor with a rumbling tummy, should ensure neither blood sugar nor digestion disrupt your shut-eye.

3. Patience makes for a perfect night's sleep

A study undertaken by the Journal of Clinical Sleep Medicine made an important discovery - the sleep-improving effects of exercise may take a while to kick in. The participants of the study group found their sleep hadn't changed much following eight weeks of exercise but fast forward to sixteen weeks, however, and their sleep patterns were reported as 'greatly improved', with the exercising group sleeping up to 1.25 hours more than their non-exercising counterparts.

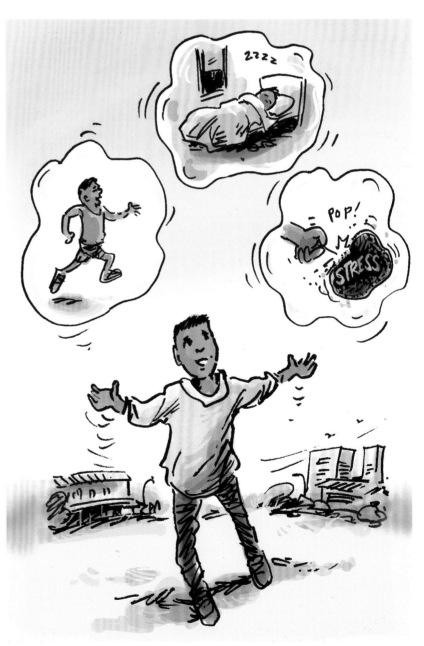

Patience prescription

Try varying your activity so that your exercise regime is easier to stick to while you wait for its sleep-enhancing benefits to kick in. Try that new dance class or break up those cardio sessions with a weekly yoga class. Ensuring you include all components of fitness in your routine will affect sleep in different ways: flexibility sessions will help you unwind, while cardio and lifting weights may help you de-stress.

4. Mornings matter

After a less fitful sleep? Try a morning workout. North Carolina's Appalachian State University conducted a small study whereby individuals all undertook moderate intensity, 30-minute workouts first thing in the morning at 7am, at lunchtime at 1pm and then at 7pm in the evening.

Researchers monitored their sleep following all exercise times and found that participants woke less during the night following a morning workout than when they'd exercised in the afternoon or evening. The exercisers also experienced a reduction in blood pressure both during the day and at night.

Early bird word

If you're keen to try the early morning workout as a means of improving your sleep, make sure you have everything in place to make that exercise session happen. Eat right the night before (not too much so your sleep's affected by your digestion working overtime; not so little your rumbling tummy wakes you) and plan an easy-to-digest, pre-exercise snack for the morning. Prepare your kit in advance, plan a good playlist to get you in the mood and take a chance on a java jolt as you have the rest of the day for its effects to wear off.

5. Less stress equals better quality sleep

If you often find yourself heading to bed with the weight of the world on your shoulders, a workout may be just the ticket. With exercise increasing your body's production of endorphins, your feel good neurotransmitters, you'll invariably finish any exercise session feeling more positive, optimistic and relaxed.

Pretty much all forms of exercise should help ease the day's stresses and strains but many find the rhythmic, repetitive motion of many types of cardiovascular training (think running, rowing or elliptical) work particularly well, while the slowing of pace that accompanies stretching workouts such as yoga will relax both body and mind.

Stress-free suggestion

Taking time out to head to the gym or hit the tarmac may not be the easiest thing in the world when you're stressed, but try and make it a habit nonetheless. Schedule these sessions in your diary as you would any other appointment and if necessary, get an exercise buddy on board so you have double the resolve.

22 January 2020

Just how much do sleep and exercise matter?

Could sleep and exercise be key to easing the global burden of mental health?

By Jennifer Newson Ph.D.

When it comes to our mental wellbeing, we are not an island. What's going on inside our heads is a direct reflection of what's going on around us. We see this clearly in the mental and emotional strain caused by global events such as the COVID-19 pandemic, but there are many other ways that life's adversities can chip away at our mental wellbeing or trigger serious mental illness. Within scientific circles, research has also regularly highlighted how life experience can influence both the onset and the trajectory of mental health disorders, emphasizing how important it is that clinicians consider a patient's life situation when making a diagnosis or when choosing a therapeutic intervention.

On the other side of the coin, the close connection between mental wellbeing and life experience provides a window for making changes that can directly or indirectly benefit our mental health and wellbeing. Although we don't always have full control over the adversities and traumas that we face, there are other aspects of how we live our lives that provide opportunities for self-management of our own mental wellbeing.

The role of sleep and exercise in mental health

The importance of sleep is undisputed and over the last few decades, there have been a whole host of scientific studies that have tried to explain why sleep is so important not just to our bodies, but also to our brains. On top of this, there's also lots of research demonstrating the grave consequences of poor sleep quality and sleep deprivation on both our mental and physical health. This includes things like performing more poorly on cognitively demanding activities and a heightened emotional and physical response to stressful situations, neither of which is helpful as we all try to navigate hectic daily schedules. And although scientists are still trying to understand the relationship between sleep and mental health, there is likely to be a negative feedback loop where poor sleep contributes to poorer mental wellbeing, which in turn leads to poorer sleep.

Similarly, when it comes to exercise then there are hundreds of scientific articles trying to understand how keeping physically active impacts our mental health and wellbeing. And while the benefits are hard to deny given the amount of supportive evidence, scientists still aren't clear about the size of the benefit that exercise brings, nor how this benefit varies across different types of exercise and across individuals who perhaps present different mental health profiles.

Relationship between sleep & mental wellbeing

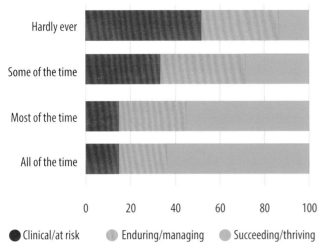

● Clinical/at risk   Enduring/managing   Succeeding/thriving

Relationship between exercise & mental wellbeing

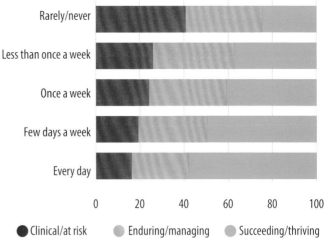

● Clinical/at risk   Enduring/managing   Succeeding/thriving

In general, I get as much sleep as I need:

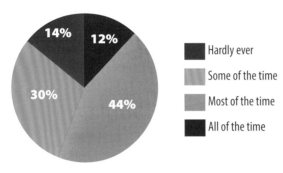

- Hardly ever
- Some of the time
- Most of the time
- All of the time

How often do you exercise
(30 minutes or more)

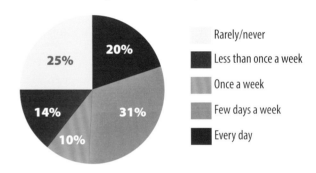

- Rarely/never
- Less than once a week
- Once a week
- Few days a week
- Every day

Source: Sapian Labs

Measuring sleep and exercise in the Mental Health Million Project

The Mental Health Million Project, which uses a free and anonymous assessment of mental wellbeing with a tool called the MHQ, tracks the ongoing mental health of the population to build a global map of mental wellbeing and help generate a better understanding of the drivers. To date, tens of thousands of people have already taken the MHQ.

So what can the Mental Health Million Project tell us about how sleep and exercise relate to a population's mental wellbeing? And how we are faring along these dimensions?

The data we've collected so far tells us that a full 50% of those who hardly ever got enough sleep have or are at risk for a clinical disorder (red on the bar chart above). Contrast that to only 14% of those who get enough sleep all the time. In other words, people who rarely get enough sleep are almost four times as likely to experience mental health challenges.

That should be enough to send everyone to bed on time. Yet the data indicate that only 12% get enough sleep all of the time and almost half are seriously sleep-deprived.

Similarly, when we take a look at the frequency of exercise, 40% of those who report that they rarely or never exercise had or were at risk for a clinical disorder (red in the graph, top right). In contrast, only 18% of those who exercised 30 mins or more every day were at risk for a clinical disorder. In other words, non-exercisers are twice as likely to be experiencing serious mental health challenges.

Yet we also find that half of those who have taken part are not regular exercisers and a full quarter rarely or never exercise.

With this kind of profound difference, it's entirely possible that mandating everyone to the gym and then straight to bed could have a significant impact on the burden of mental health. Yet more insights are needed into the direction of cause and effect, the nature of symptoms associated with poor sleep and exercise, and differences by factors such as age and gender.

Identifying the mental health challenges faced by different populations across the globe is an important step in being able to address them effectively. It is our hope that creating a data map of these challenges will not only help from a global surveillance perspective but will also improve understanding of the role of social and economic factors and life experiences, informing therapeutic intervention and policy decisions. Stay tuned for more insights from the project in future posts.

20 November 2020

Time to tackle the physical activity gender gap

2019 might well be the year of women's sport. While coverage has long been overshadowed by the male leagues, viewing opportunities and public engagement has been growing. Public excitement perhaps peaked during the Women's Football World Cup, with television audiences across the world increased by millions on previous years. As female athletes challenge inequalities over pay and investment and shift social expectations, could their example be used to tackle the gender gap in physical activity in the wider population?

Insufficient physical activity is a leading risk factor for non-communicable diseases and can also negatively affect mental health and quality of life. WHO recognises physical inactivity as a serious and growing public health problem and aims to reduce it by 10% by 2025. An analysis published in The Lancet Global Health, in 2018, found that more than a quarter of adults globally are insufficiently physically active. Across most countries, women are less active than men (global average of 31·7% for inactive women vs 23·4% for inactive men). Policies that tackle the gender gap in physical activity could therefore have a substantial impact on overall population health.

The barriers to women's involvement in sports are numerous and complex. The physical activity gap between boys and girls begins early. A report from Sport England found that girls aged 3–11 years experienced less enjoyment from being physically active and less confidence in their sporting ability than boys as they got older. Children's exposure to narrow gender norms around boys' versus girls' activities and a failure to adapt the types of sports offered can instil this lack of enjoyment and body confidence, and in turn shape attitudes to physical activity into adulthood. Indeed, many women are put off by certain physical activities over concerns about stereotypes, because of insecurities around body image, or feeling constrained by cultural acceptability. Women and girls' sport generally receives less investment at the grassroots level—including access to equipment, transport, and coaching, and to safe and welcoming facilities. Women still often play the lead role in child care and managing households—for many, in addition to paid work—which means they generally have less leisure time.

Addressing the gender gap in physical activity could therefore start with better access, investment, and shifting sociocultural norms. Changes to the built environment and providing exercise facilities to the public is one approach, and some evidence suggests that more walkable cities had lower gender gaps in physical activity. However, built environment is not the whole picture. The study by Claire Nightingale and colleagues in this issue of The Lancet Public Health found that residents who moved to a neighbourhood created along active design principles (the former London 2012 Olympic and Paralympic Games Athletes' Village) showed no significant increase in their average physical activity. Changes in urban environment should probably be accompanied by community and behavioural public health interventions.

One example of a promising intervention has been the This Girl Can campaign in England. Launched in 2015, the

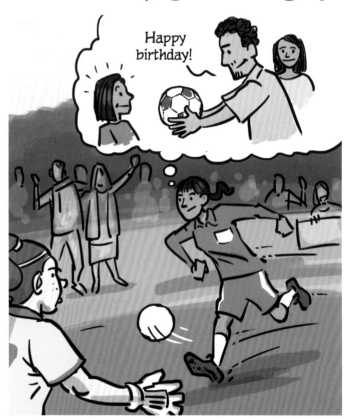

multimedia campaign focused on projecting an inclusive, positive message about physical activity and could have helped an estimated 3 million women and girls become more physically active. However, such campaigns still face the challenge of widening participation to reach women from low-income and from ethnic minority backgrounds. Adapting interventions and opportunities to these groups will be important. It is also unclear to what extent such a campaign might be adapted to low-income or middle-income countries – and this should be the focus of future research.

The universality of sport offers an opportunity to challenge social and cultural norms on a large scale and narrow the gender gap. By making female athletic success more visible, girls and their parents can aspire for them to be professional athletes or simply to take part in whatever physical activity they enjoy. A greater audience for women's professional sport could mean more investment in grassroots and crucially, visibility of women at all sporting levels.

Ultimately, if current trends continue, the 2025 global physical activity target of a 10% relative reduction in insufficient physical activity will not be met. Multi-sectoral approaches to increase physical activity need to be prioritised urgently. Public health professionals and policy makers should capitalise on moments like the Women's World Cup to encourage and support all to be physically active. It can't be a missed opportunity.

22 July 2019

How Covid is widening the gender gap: women and children activity levels set back

Gap to men had closed significantly before Covid but after six months of lockdown, only a quarter of women are remaining regularly active.

By Jeremy Wilson, chief sports reporter

The gender gap for women in sport has widened during the devastating Covid-19 pandemic, according to a raft of new research which has also confirmed the sector's worst fears over how the crisis will impact children.

The data, which is separately published by Sport England and the Youth Sport Trust and can be revealed by *Telegraph Women's Sport*, shows how, after six months of lockdown restrictions, only a quarter of women are remaining regularly active.

The gap to men, which had closed significantly before Covid following initiatives such as Sport England's 'This Girl Can' campaign, peaked at 10 per cent early in the pandemic, but has since stabilised at around five per cent. Women were found to be more anxious about going out to exercise, more affected by caring responsibilities, comparatively worse off financially and more affected by the reduction in group activities such as exercise classes.

The visibility of elite women's sport has also been disproportionately reduced after governing bodies prioritised the return of more lucrative men's competition.

'I'm positive about the overall trajectory of women's sport, but my fear is that we will be taking a giant leap backwards because of this year,' said Chrissie Wellington, the four-time world Ironman champion and Parkrun's global lead for health and well-being.

Particularly alarming is the early data this term from schools which, despite the need to get children active following their March closures, have reduced extra-curricular activities. According to the teachers surveyed by the Youth Sports Trust, half of schools were providing fewer than 30 minutes of daily activity time for children, including 12 per cent who said that there were no active minutes at all.

Just three per cent of secondary schools said that they would be offering more PE this term, despite respectively 73 per cent and 49 per cent of teachers having identified 'low physical fitness' and 'mental well-being, including anxiety and fear' as an issue in returning pupils. All previous research has also shown that girls are disproportionately affected by a crisis of inactivity.

'What we have feared most has become a reality, children's lives have been disrupted by the pandemic and their usual

Women and girls' activity levels

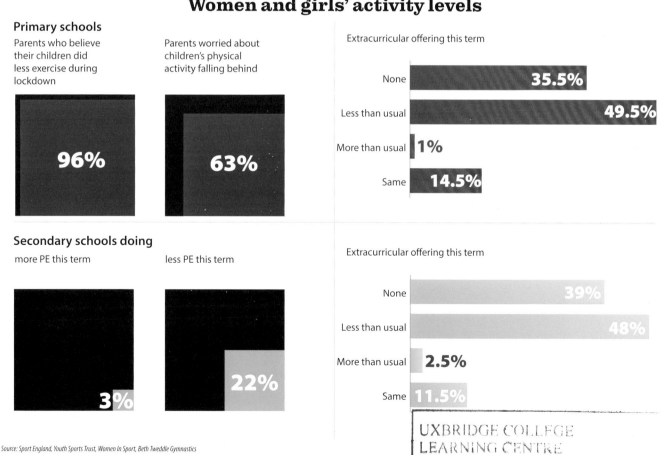

Primary schools

Parents who believe their children did less exercise during lockdown

96%

Parents worried about children's physical activity falling behind

63%

Extracurricular offering this term

- None **35.5%**
- Less than usual **49.5%**
- More than usual **1%**
- Same **14.5%**

Secondary schools doing

more PE this term

3%

less PE this term

22%

Extracurricular offering this term

- None **39%**
- Less than usual **48%**
- More than usual **2.5%**
- Same **11.5%**

Source: Sport England, Youth Sports Trust, Women In Sport, Beth Tweddle Gymnastics

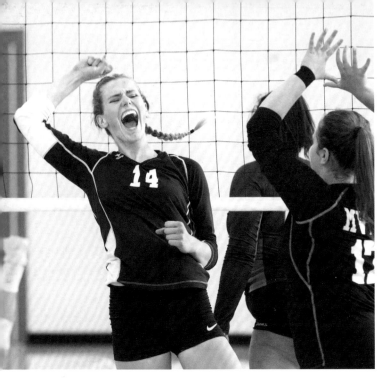

play and activity habits inhibited,' said Ali Oliver, the chief executive of the Youth Sports Trust.

'Now they return to school, we are seeing all sorts of issues present themselves from anxiety and depression to low physical fitness and self-confidence. The well-being of our children has to be a national priority.'

Industry leaders and experts have also called for:

♦ A government rescue package to ensure that community sport and activity survives the pandemic.

♦ Increased visibility of women's sport.

♦ Physical activity and well-being to be given the same priority as academic achievement in schools.

♦ A debate over the trade-off between curtailing sports and the long-term health impacts of reduced activities.

♦ A national push to get more women and girls coaching as well as participating.

The year had started from a point of relative momentum. The number of women deemed 'active', defined as 150 weekly minutes or more, was up to 61 per cent. And the gap to men had narrowed to only 3.9 per cent. Then came lockdown and, says Lisa O'Keefe, Sport England's insight director, 'overnight we suddenly saw this massive disruption and impact'.

The gender gap peaked during the first week of lockdown data and those deemed 'active' by the criteria of at least 30 minutes per day, five days a week, has been respectively 30 per cent of men and 25 per cent of women across the past three weeks.

It suggests a stark overall reduction across genders since before Covid-19, although O'Keefe stresses one potentially crucial statistic. With the Government consistently promoting activity even at the height of lockdown, 70 per cent of women do say that it is 'more important than ever to be active'. Increases in running, cycling and walking were recorded, but also particular gender barriers. Women were always far more likely to attend fitness classes and so severe limitations on choice have had a disproportionate impact and, with Covid-19 spreading, they were more reluctant than men to leave home to exercise.

Time was also a major factor. Almost two-thirds of men reported having time to be active against just over half of women and, according to a separate study by Women in Sport, almost a third of women could not prioritise exercise during lockdown because they had too much to do for others. O'Keefe believes that the industry's challenge is to match an enhanced desire to be active with suitable opportunity and inspiration.

'The conditions that have been brought about by the pandemic have, in some cases, supercharged existing barriers and anxieties,' she said. 'It is more important than ever that active women and girls are visible and celebrated.'

Schools are already seeing the physical and mental impacts on children, but Government guidance on social distancing, changing rooms, cleaning and maintaining set 'bubbles', as well as reduced and staggered lunchtimes, wet weather

Return to school activity

Active minutes for children in average school day

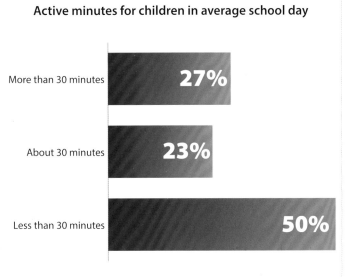

More than 30 minutes — **27%**

About 30 minutes — **23%**

Less than 30 minutes — **50%**

What issues have emerged as children have returned to school?

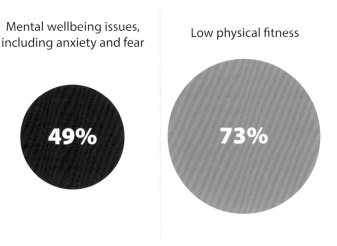

Mental wellbeing issues, including anxiety and fear — **49%**

Low physical fitness — **73%**

Source: Sport England, Youth Sports Trust, Women In Sport, Beth Tweddle Gymnastics

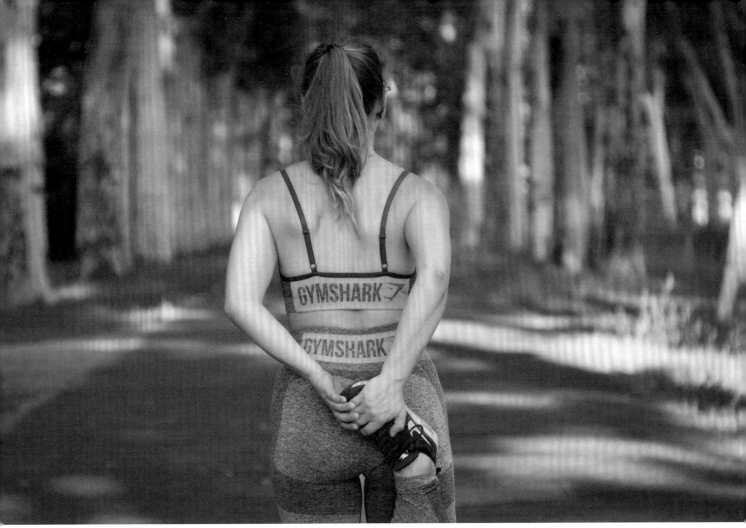

and staff shortages, are disrupting opportunities. Between 80 and 90 per cent of schools are offering either no extra-curricular sports activities or less than they previously would.

'Our insight reveals that many schools are struggling with the confidence to resume, or do not see it as a priority in relation to other subjects – with the challenge greatest in secondary schools, where over a fifth are offering less PE than before Covid,' Oliver said.

Some of the Youth Sport Trust's anecdotal feedback from teachers has included the description of the new school day as 'very sedentary' and children feeling like 'caged animals' after six months away.

Stephanie Hilborne, the chief executive of Women in Sport, has urged the Government and schools to ensure that girls are not now marginalised.

'Women and girls have borne the emotional brunt of this pandemic and one thing we owe them is the equal right to space in the playground, to kick or throw a ball, to run about and shout, to be carefree and high spirited,' she said.

A desire to promote physical activity is at least evident. The charity Greenhouse Sports, which provides sports coaching, has reported unprecedented interest from schools in its programmes while Beth Tweddle, the former world champion gymnast, has already had 450 primary schools sign up for her free 10-week physical literacy programme.

Tweddle wants PE prioritised and believes that the key to inspiring girls is working with them to discover what offering they want. 'There is a sport for everyone – it's finding what you engage with,' she says.

It is a mantra echoed by Wellington, who says that Parkrun's phenomenal success across genders is founded simply on breaking down barriers to participation and delivery. Asked how to inspire girls in sport, she said: 'We need to listen and stop imposing solutions. We have to meet women and girls where they are and work with the reality of their lives.'

With Parkrun still tentatively planning its return next month, Wellington also highlighted the unintended health consequences of lockdown and how the most disadvantaged communities were being hit hardest.

'I feel strongly that a debate needs to be had about the long-term impacts of these [lockdown] measures,' she said. 'There are deep and persistent health and well-being inequalities, and the Covid pandemic has compounded and exacerbated them. We need resilient communities built on interaction, health and well-being.' As well as more than half a million female Parkrun runners and walkers, there are also almost 100,000 volunteers. Maintaining and increasing community sport's base of volunteers is, according to Mark Gannon, UK Coaching's chief executive, also critical. 'Schools will be so preoccupied with trying to catch up academically that community sport is more important now than ever,' he said. 'My fear is that women and girls' sport could go back 10 years. It's had such fantastic momentum – and that is something we must not now lose.'

24 September 2020

We simply cannot rely on school PE lessons to provide enough exercise for children

Even at the best of times, schools struggle to provide pupils with adequate physical education.

By Oliver Brown, Chief sports writer

As the children of the pandemic prepare once more to have their escapist joys cruelly curtailed, the Government needs to be aware of a crucial false premise in its own logic. By decreeing that children who spend their daylight hours indoors in classes of 30 must not join their friends at weekends for games of seven-a-side, it implies an assumption that schools can still furnish all the physical education required. Such faith, alas, is sadly misplaced. For even at the best of times, the PE provision in the National Curriculum is far from adequate, let alone when the nation is plunged into fresh paralysis just as the nights draw in.

Already, pupils are being taught fewer hours of PE than they were a decade ago. Last year, research by Sport England highlighted how 80 per cent were failing to do the 60 minutes of daily physical exercise recommended by the chief medical officer. The precedent for this oversight is all too often set in schools, where the hours for PE are typically half those for maths or English. So much, then,

for the Government's previous insistence that children's physical vitality should be accorded the same importance as their literacy or numeracy. According to the Youth Sport Trust, one in four schools have reduced PE's presence on the timetable since 2017, a situation about to be gruesomely exacerbated by a second lockdown.

When the schools shut in March, many parents contrived novel means to keep their children active amid the monotony, from setting up trampolines in the back garden to hooking them up to the YouTube wisdom of Joe Wicks. It helped that the Prime Minister had delivered his initial stay-at-home message just three days after the spring equinox, and that the first lockdown's interminable extensions were tempered in May by the sunniest month on record. The scenario this time is altogether grimmer. The Stygian gloom of November compels children towards a screen rather than to a couple of rain-lashed laps of the park. The Government's response is simply to enable this slide towards indolence by thwarting every form of exercise that they can enjoy together.

Activity levels have fallen

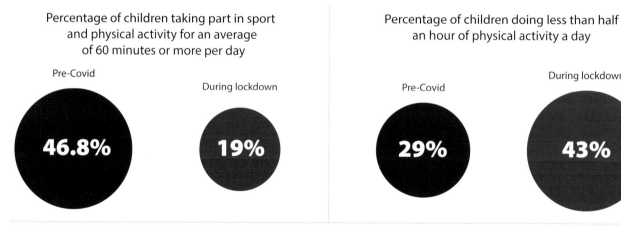

Percentage of children taking part in sport and physical activity for an average of 60 minutes or more per day

Pre-Covid: 46.8%
During lockdown: 19%

Percentage of children doing less than half an hour of physical activity a day

Pre-Covid: 29%
During lockdown: 43%

Percentage of children who did nothing to stay active in lockdown
7%

Percentage of children who said they were less active than normal
31%

Percentage of children who were more active
13%

Source: Sport England lockdown survey and Youth Sports Trust

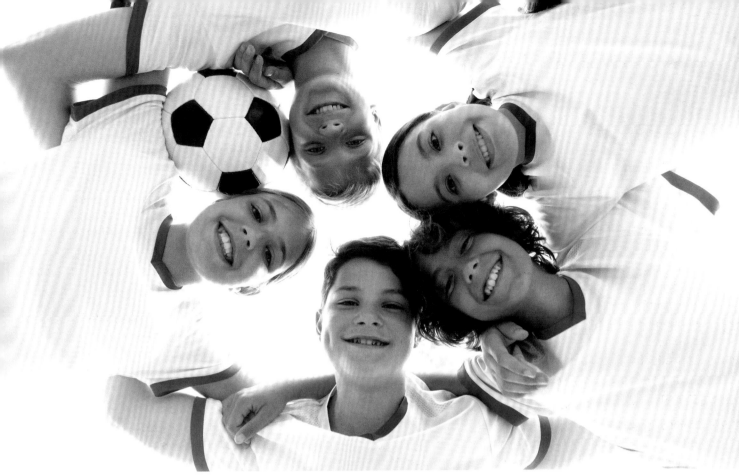

A treatise could be written on all that has happened to Boris Johnson between March and November 2020, but his failure to fight for PE gives one telling illustration of the dwindling courage of his convictions. As mayor of London, he was so bullish about fulfilling the 2012 Olympics' promise to 'inspire a generation' that he called for children to have compulsory competitive games every morning. 'It is time to begin a campaign – a crusade – for sport in schools,' he wrote in this newspaper in 2015. 'Daily organised sport would be fantastic for children's concentration, for their intellectual performance, for their health, and ultimately for their longevity.'

In the 15 months that he has had to enact these laudable sentiments into law, the gap between rhetoric and reality has been glaringly exposed. In his 15-minute press conference speech last Saturday night, a PM who once spoke of children's physical wellbeing as essential to the health of the nation neglected even to mention this theme, despite knowing the devastation his latest restrictions would inflict.

In Lockdown One, children's physical outlets were sustained by a mixture of benign weather and parental intuition. Even though the schools are open throughout Lockdown Two, there is no such safety net. For a start, the politicians' crowd-pleasing of PE is still not reflected in the curriculum. Although there is a stated guideline of two hours' PE per week, it is still not mandatory, undermining the World Health Organisation's argument that children should have at least three weekly exercise sessions to maintain a healthy body. In Singapore, two hours' worth is the minimum. In Sweden, for 11- to 13-year-olds, it is closer to four. For the UK

not to be among the global leaders in this department is a national embarrassment.

The elements present another obstacle that seems to have escaped the Government's attention. Just as there is an apparent obliviousness to the idea that women will not feel perfectly safe exercising alone after dark, there is a disregard of how children's exercise patterns, just like everything else in the UK, follow a seasonal pattern. It is scarcely a coincidence that activity levels among under-18s are lowest when the days grow shorter, colder and wetter.

School cross-country runs in the teeth of an Arctic gale are seldom recalled with much fondness. But they threaten soon to be all that is left. *The Telegraph*'s Keep Kids Active campaign is one that recognises the physical and mental health crisis that is about to be unleashed. It is not too late for the Government to mitigate the damage, and it can begin by understanding that schools will never meet the nation's PE needs on their own.

2 November 2020

Exercise and mental health – the benefits of exercise on mental health

Exercise plays a large part in physical and mental health. Getting up and active can have some great benefits for your general wellbeing, and luckily, you don't have to start a rigorous training plan. Instead, small amounts of activity, from taking the stairs to walking to the bus stop, can help.

The benefits of exercise on mental health

Exercise is shown to have many benefits including energy increase, self-esteem boost, better sleep, promoting relaxation, and stronger resilience. One of the biggest advantages of exercise is the stimulation of chemicals in the brain which can promote growth of new brain cells, prevent age related cognitive decline and aid concentration. Exercise releases endorphins, the so-called 'feel good' chemical, known for boosting moods.

This is not to say exercise will solve any mental health symptoms. Instead, exercise is likely to alleviate some of the symptoms, even if only for a short while. If you are concerned about your wellbeing, speak to a professional.

Here are some specific ways in which exercise benefits mental health:

Exercise and depression

Exercise can be prescribed as treatment by GPs for a variety of conditions including mild to moderate depression. Alternative treatments include medication or psychological therapy. Through exercising, it has been found changes in the brain occur such as activity patterns promoting feelings of calm and well-being. Additionally, the release of endorphins from exercise is known to elevate moods.

Exercise and anxiety

Exercise relieves tension and stress as well as boosting physical energy. When experiencing feelings of anxiety, exercising can be a good way to lessen stress, not through distracting oneself, but through focussing on the body and its power. Focus on sensation of feet hitting the ground, breathing patterns, and how the body is moving. Exercise can generally help increase mindfulness and allow one to regain control.

Exercise and ADHD

Those who experience ADHD may benefit from exercising to reduce symptoms. Getting active can improve concentration, motivation and memory as well as boost the brain chemicals dopamine, norepinephrine and serotonin, all affecting focus and attention.

Exercise and physical health

If suffering from physical aliments, exercise can help. Exercising can reduce the risk of heart disease, stroke, diabetes, obesity, and many other health issues. Through sustained active changes towards physical health, mental health will likely improve too.

If you haven't exercised in a while or have health conditions, check with your doctor before beginning. Take care to avoid injury or negative emotional responses to exercise.

Short term endorphins may feel good, but exercise must be regular for longer term effects to take hold.

Benefits of exercise on mental health – how to get started

As aforementioned, don't jump straight into vigorous exercise. Here are some top tips for getting started with exercising.

Routine

Having a routine can help sleep and eating patterns, as well as ensure you stick to your exercise. The government advises adults do 150 minutes of moderate intensity activity each week – as simple as a 25 minute walk each day. Maybe make walking the children to and from school part of your routine. Or a morning jog. Or an evening cycle class three times a week. Find a way to fit exercise around your life.

Start small

There is little point in setting unattainable goals and giving up at the first hurdle. Instead set manageable goals that may still slightly challenge and motivate you. Why not try a monthly challenge? You can choose from a range of goal distances and complete it over the course of a month at your own pace.

Enjoy exercise

Try a few different methods of exercise including classes, swimming, and team sport to see what you enjoy. If you don't enjoy it, you are less likely to continue exercising. Even gardening or walking the dog counts!

Exercise with friends

Exercising with a friend, or multiple, has many benefits! Whether you are nervous to go alone, feel motivated by someone else, or simply fancy having a chat while you exercise, having someone else there is great. Read our blog post about the benefits of exercising with a friend to find out more.

Get comfortable

If you don't feel comfortable going to a gym, work out somewhere else – there are plenty of ways to get fit without a gym. If you want to wear certain clothes, to feel comfortable, wear them. Take steps that make you feel at ease, so you feel happy exercising.

Go outside

If possible, exercise outside from time to time. Evidence suggests doing physical activity in an outdoor/green environment has greater positive effects on wellbeing compared to activity indoors. Grab a friend, your dog, or just your music and head to your local park, you may be

New #TimeTogether campaign to get teenage girls and mums physically active

A new national campaign aims to bridge the physical activity gender gap between women and men by empowering daughters and mums to get active together.

By Tom Walker

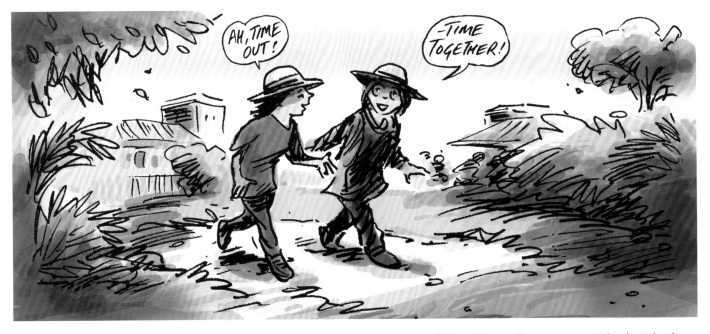

L aunched by Women in Sport, #TimeTogether looks to help daughters and mums discover new ways of spending time with each other – by inspiring them to dance, walk, climb, swim and play sport together.

Currently, only 42 per cent of teenage girls meet physical activity guidelines and just under a third of girls (32 per cent) are inactive, engaging in less than an average of 30 minutes' activity per day.

The figures, from Sport England's Active Lives survey, also shows that 65 per cent of men are likely to be active, in comparison to 61 per cent of women

Meanwhile, Women in Sport's own studies show that mums are often reluctant to allocate time for themselves to be active, with 32 per cent of women saying that they couldn't prioritise exercise during lockdown as they had too much to do for others.

The #TimeTogether campaign will see host of organisations – including Places Leisure, Our Parks and This Mum Runs – offering activity ideas for mums and daughters across the UK to try.

Those getting active are then encouraged to share their experiences using the #TimeTogether hashtag across social media platforms.

'Our research has shown that teenage girls cherish alone time with their mum and view their relationship as a "safe space" without any fear of judgement,' said Stephanie Hilborne, CEO of Women in Sport.

'This campaign provides an opportunity for them to find their judgement free space together, get active, and discover the joy, fun and well-being benefits of exercise.

'Our insights show that girls in their teens feel burdened by school work and social expectations, and at the same time the lives of their mothers are often fraught with growing pressures of work and providing emotional support and care for relatives.

'We want every mother and every daughter to feel they have permission to take time out to have fun outside and be active. There has rarely been a more important time for such special mutual support and to be active together than in this pandemic.'

3 November 2020

Physical activity can help children catch up on missed work

New research shows students and teachers report physical activity can improve pupils' mood, confidence and schoolwork.

Physically active children report improvements in their schoolwork, behaviour and mental health, according to new research from Sheffield Hallam University.

The study, conducted on more than 60,000 students and 4,000 teachers, was part of our Secondary Teacher Training (STT) programme and surveyed their attitudes to work, physical and mental health.

This research shows that helping children and young people to get active during school can play a vital role in helping them catch up work missed during the coronavirus (Covid-19) pandemic, and in supporting their mental health.

The STT programme is a collaboration between us, the Activity Alliance, the Association for Physical Education and the Youth Sport Trust, and provides funding and access to

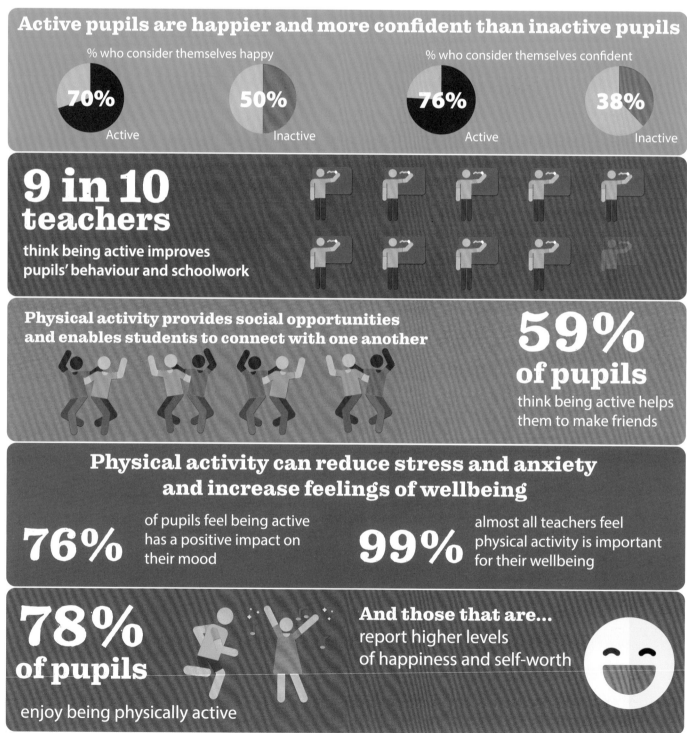

Active pupils are happier and more confident than inactive pupils

% who consider themselves happy

70% Active

50% Inactive

% who consider themselves confident

76% Active

38% Inactive

9 in 10 teachers think being active improves pupils' behaviour and schoolwork

Physical activity provides social opportunities and enables students to connect with one another

59% of pupils think being active helps them to make friends

Physical activity can reduce stress and anxiety and increase feelings of wellbeing

76% of pupils feel being active has a positive impact on their mood

99% almost all teachers feel physical activity is important for their wellbeing

78% of pupils enjoy being physically active

And those that are... report higher levels of happiness and self-worth

* Based on a study by Sheffield Hallam University of 62,453 pupils and 4,458 members of staff for Sport England's Secondary Teacher Training programme

Source: Sport England

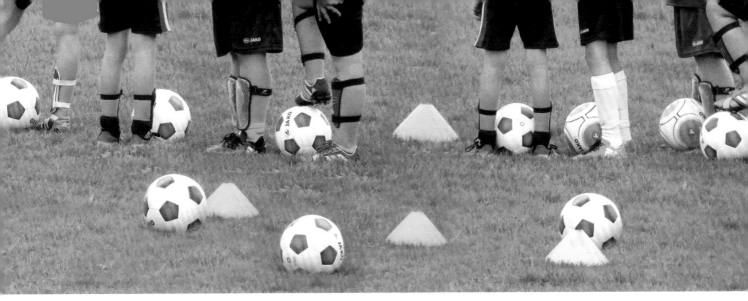

professional development opportunities for PE teachers across the country.

Part of the programme was this research, which shows 92% of staff believe being physically active helps with school work, and that 91% of students report feeling that physical activity can improve their mental and physical health.

'When schools were closed, we know that children found it harder to get active and did less activity than normal,' said our chief executive, Tim Hollingsworth.

'Now that they are back open, we have a fantastic opportunity to help them reengage with both sport and exercise – and this new research tells us it's not only great for their physical health, it boosts their mental health, supports good behaviour, and academic achievement too.

'Teachers are under pressure right now and we hope we can relieve some of that by delivering with our partners free support for schools in how to engage students with physical activity.

'It's based on our knowledge of what it takes to build physical literacy – that they are more likely to take part if activity is enjoyable, if there's choice, and they are involved in the design of opportunities.

'It will also help staff to take a whole school approach to healthy lifestyles, creating opportunities before, after and throughout the school day.'

The activity levels of many children and young people have reduced significantly from pre-lockdown, with a third of children reporting the absence of school had a major impact on their ability to be active.

Happier and more confident

Other findings from the study include:

♦ Active students are happier (70% vs 50%) and more confident to try sport (76% vs 38%) than inactive students.

♦ Young people report that being physically active improves their mood (71%), behaviour (55%) and schoolwork (49%).

♦ The vast majority of staff agree with this, with 93% reporting feeling that being active benefits pupil behaviour and 92% reporting they feel it has positive effects on schoolwork.

♦ Activity provides social opportunities and enables students to connect with one another, with 59% agreeing it helps them to make friends.

♦ Physical activity has the potential to reduce stress and anxiety by providing routine and structure and increasing feelings of wellbeing: 76% of students and 99% of staff feel that being active has a positive effect on their mood.

♦ Students who are active report higher levels of happiness and self-worth.

♦ 87% of staff feel that being physically active has a positive impact on the school environment (ethos, values, culture, identity).

♦ The majority of students surveyed (78%) enjoy being physically active.

With schools now reopened, the programme can help with simple things such as helping schools to offer more choice in how to be active and building activity across the school day.

Coming with the new research is free support to help schools include physical activity into lessons, adapt PE to make sure more students enjoy it and build in active travel to and from school.

The research is particularly timely, with today being the start of Walk to School Week and schools encouraging students to build active minutes into their day before they even get to school.

'At Telford Priory School we decided to involve students in establishing our priorities for our PE curriculum,' said Telford Priory School deputy headteacher Imran Iqbal.

'The Secondary Teacher Training programme has helped to support our teachers deliver enjoyable sport for all abilities, which has helped create a monumental shift in reaching students who traditionally sat on the periphery of PE lessons.

'The benefits of keeping students safely active has never been more important than it is now.'

5 October 2020

Light activity may improve mental health for teenagers

'Teenagers who sit for hours a day are more likely to get depression at 18'
reports the Mail Online.

It's been known for some time that children's activity levels go down as they get older, and this seems to be happening more in recent years. The numbers of teenagers with depression have also been rising.

Researchers tracked the activity levels of 4,257 teenagers aged 12, 14 and 16. They then tested them for symptoms of depression at age 18. During the study, average levels of light activity, such as slow walking, fell. Time spent sitting or lying down increased. More time spent doing light activity at age 12 to 16 was linked to lower depression scores at age 18, while more time spent sitting still was linked to higher depression scores.

Only 1.5% of those in the study were meeting government recommendations for people aged 5 to 18 to do an hour of moderate intensity activity each day.

The researchers say it might be easier for teenagers to do more light activity than to increase the amount of moderate-to-vigorous activity they do. Even the relatively small decreases in depression scores seen in the study could have an important impact on the mental health of some young people.

Where did the story come from?

The researchers who carried out the study were from University College London and King's College London. The study was funded by the Medical Research Council, the Wellcome Trust and the University of Bristol. It was published in the peer-reviewed medical journal Lancet Psychiatry, on an open-access basis, so it is free to read online.

The study is reported with reasonable accuracy and balance by the UK media, although the limitations of the study and possible alternative explanations for the results are not explained.

What kind of research was this?

This was a cohort study. Cohort studies, like other observational studies, are good ways to look at links between risk factors (such as levels of physical activity) and outcomes (such as depression symptoms). But they cannot show that one directly causes another. There may be other factors involved.

What did the research involve?

Researchers in Bristol recruited pregnant women in 1991 to take part in a long-running study (the Avon Longitudinal Study of Parents and Children). The children born as a result of those pregnancies were followed up regularly with health checks and questionnaires.

In this study, researchers looked at groups of teenagers who had at least 1 measure of physical activity taken by a device called an accelerometer at age 12 (2,486 teens), 14

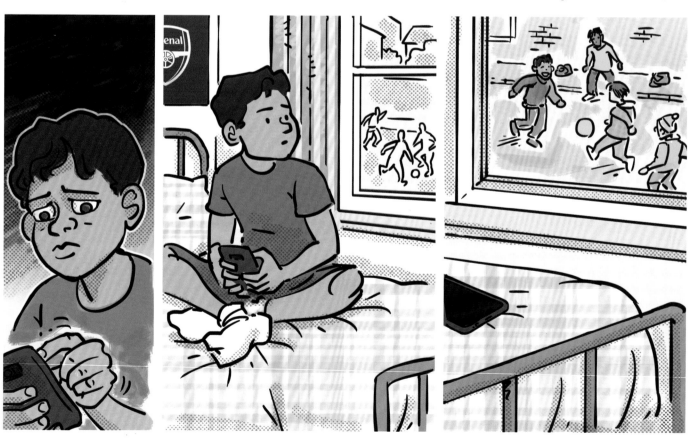

(1,938 teens) or 16 (1,220 teens), and had been tested for symptoms of depression at age 18 (4,257 teens) using the CIS-R depression score computer assessment. They analysed the results for links between depression symptom scores and:

♦ total physical activity at age 12, 14, or 16

♦ sedentary time (time spent sitting or lying down)

♦ light activity (such as slow walking)

♦ moderate to vigorous activity (such as running or sports)

They took account of factors including their sex, ethnic background, social class, signs of depression at age 12, IQ, any history of serious mental illness in the parents and parental education level. They also adjusted figures for the amount of time the teenagers wore the accelerometer.

What were the basic results?

The researchers found teenagers spent about an hour and a half (93 minutes) longer each day sitting still or lying down at age 16 compared to age 12. They spent an hour and 20 minutes (81 minutes) less time each day doing light physical activity at age 16 compared with age 12. Time spent doing moderate to vigorous physical activity remained about the same, although it was at a low level (around 20 minutes) from the start.

About 17% to 18% of teenagers had symptom scores that might mean they had depression at age 18.

When researchers looked at time spent sitting still or lying down, they found teenagers who spent more time sitting down had higher depression scores, while teenagers who spent more time doing light activity had lower scores:

♦ each additional hour per day spent sitting still at age 12 to 16 was linked to an 11% to 8% increase in depression symptom score at age 18 (incidence rate ratio (IRR) age 12: 1.11, 95% confidence interval (CI) 1.05 to 1.18; IRR age 14: 1.08, 95% CI 1.01 to 1.15; IRR age 16: 1.11, 95% CI 1.02 to 1.21)

♦ each additional hour per day spent doing light activity at age 12 to 16 was linked to an 11% to 8% decrease in depression symptom score at age 18 (IRR age 12: 0.90, 95% CI 0.85 to 0.96; IRR age 14: 0.92, 95% CI 0.86 to 0.99; IRR age 16: 0.89, 95% CI 0.81 to 0.97)

The teenagers' moderate-to-vigorous physical activity levels did not seem strongly linked to depression scores. This could be because too few of them were doing sufficient moderate-to-vigorous physical activity to make an impression on the results.

Spending more time, overall, doing physical activity was also linked to lower depression scores.

How did the researchers interpret the results?

The researchers said: 'The displacement of sedentary behaviour with light activity in young people warrants more direct and specific consideration in physical activity guidelines and public health interventions aimed at reducing the prevalence of depression.' They called for schools to encourage 'standing lessons, increasing active travel time between classes, or promoting lightly active hobbies such as playing an instrument and painting.'

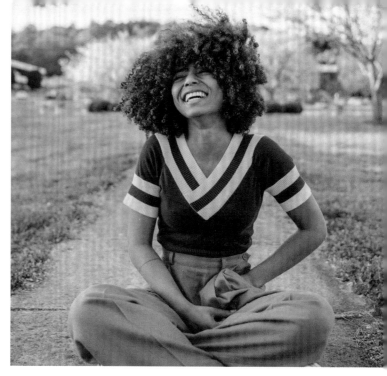

Conclusion

The link between physical activity and mental health has been investigated for some time. But this is the first study to have looked at accelerometer-measured activity – including light activity – in teenagers and the link to mental health.

Physical activity, whether that's doing household chores or training to run a marathon, has consistently been shown to benefit physical and mental health. A study that shows even light activity may benefit teenager's mental health is therefore welcome.

However, there are some limitations to the study. Physical activity and mental health may both be linked to other factors, such as the environment in which children live, their physical health, social support and the amount of time they spend using a screen. For example, a child who does not have a safe space to be active outdoors may be more likely to spend a lot of time indoors, sitting or lying down, and may also have poorer mental health. It is difficult to say which of these factors is most important.

Teenagers in the study also tended to drop out of physical activity monitoring as the study progressed, meaning there were more records of activity at age 12 than at age 16. This could explain why the links between depression scores and activity levels at age 12 seem stronger than at age 16. There were only 1,220 records of activity at age 16, compared with 2,486 at age 12.

Despite the limits of the study, the message that teenagers should be encouraged to be more active for the sake of their mental health is an important one. Symptoms of depression often emerge for the first time during adolescence. Efforts to stop and reverse the increasing inactivity of children and young people could have important effects on future mental health.

12 February 2020

Dieting and weight worries on rise in teens

Significantly higher numbers of Generation Z boys and girls in the UK are dieting to lose weight, and are likely to overestimate their own weight, finds a new UCL-led study.

The research, published in *JAMA Pediatrics*, found that girls who are trying to lose weight are also more likely to experience depressive symptoms than in previous years.

In 2015, 42% of 14-year-old girls and boys said they currently were trying to lose weight, compared to 30% in 2005.

Lead author Dr Francesca Solmi (UCL Psychiatry) said: 'Our findings show how the way we talk about weight, health and appearance can have profound impacts on young people's mental health, and efforts to tackle rising obesity rates may have unintended consequences.

'An increase in dieting among young people is concerning because experimental studies have found that dieting is generally ineffective in the long term at reducing body weight in adolescents, but can instead have greater impacts on mental health. We know, for instance, that dieting is a strong risk factor in the development of eating disorders.'

The research team reviewed data from 22,503 adolescents in the UK, in three different decades, who are part of different cohort studies: the British Cohort Study (of people born in 1970; data was collected in 1986), the Children of the 90s study (born 1991-92, data collected in 2005), and Millennium Cohort Study (born 2000-02, data collected in 2015).

The adolescents were all asked questions about whether they were, or had been, trying to lose weight, whether they had dieted or exercised to lose weight, whether they perceived themselves to be underweight, about the right weight or overweight (which was compared to their actual height and weight measurements), and they filled out questionnaires that gauged depressive symptoms.

The researchers found that in 2015, 44% and 60% of all participants had dieted or exercised to lose weight, respectively, compared to 38% and 7% in 1986.

The researchers say other evidence suggests that engagement in vigorous physical activity has remained relatively stable among adolescents over the past few decades.

Senior author Dr Praveetha Patalay (Centre for Longitudinal Studies and MRC Unit for Lifelong Health & Ageing, UCL) said: 'It seems that young people are exercising for different reasons than they did before – more adolescents seem to be thinking of exercise predominantly as a means to lose weight rather than exercising for fun, socialising and feeling healthy. We suspect that recent controversial calls to add 'exercise-equivalent' labels on food packaging may exacerbate this.'

While girls have consistently been more likely to diet to lose weight, the researchers found a greater increase over the years among boys, who were also becoming more likely to be trying to gain weight.

Dr Patalay said: 'Societal pressures for girls to be thin have been around for decades, but body image pressures on boys may be a more recent trend. Our findings underscore the impact that societal pressures and public health messaging around weight can have on children's health behaviours, body image and mental health.'

Both girls and boys also became more likely to over-estimate their weight from 1986 to 2005, and even more so by 2015, which the researchers say adds to their concerns that increased efforts to lose weight are not necessarily due to increased obesity rates.

The reported weight-related behaviours and weight misperception were associated with depressive symptoms, and among girls, this relationship was becoming even stronger over the three decades examined in this study. The findings could possibly be part of the explanation for increases in adolescent depressive symptoms that have been observed in recent decades.

Dr Solmi said: 'Media portrayals of thinness, the rise of the fitness industry and the advent of social media may all partly explain our results, and public health messaging around calorie restriction and exercise might also be causing unintended harm.

'Public health campaigns around obesity should consider adverse mental health effects, and ensure they avoid weight stigma. By promoting health and wellbeing, as opposed to focusing on "healthy weight", they could have positive effects on both mental and physical health.'

The study was conducted by researchers at UCL and the Universities of Edinburgh and Liverpool, and was supported by Wellcome, the National Institute for Health Research UCLH Biomedical Research Centre, the Economic and Social Research Council, the Medical Research Council and the University of Bristol.

16 November 2020

College teens shun exercise and healthy food, study finds

♦ Only one in five participants had a BMI classified as obese - but nine out of ten 16-18 year olds admit not exercising enough

♦ Three in ten did no exercise per week

♦ Eight out of ten not eating enough fruit and veg, with one in ten eating no fruit or veg at all, and half only eating 1-2 portions a day

Older teenagers may be setting a course for lifelong obesity through inactivity and poor diets, according to a new study.

Scientists at the University of Reading say the findings add to the growing evidence showing radical changes are needed to influence the health and diet of children and teenagers, as the UK government launches a new nationwide strategy to tackle obesity.

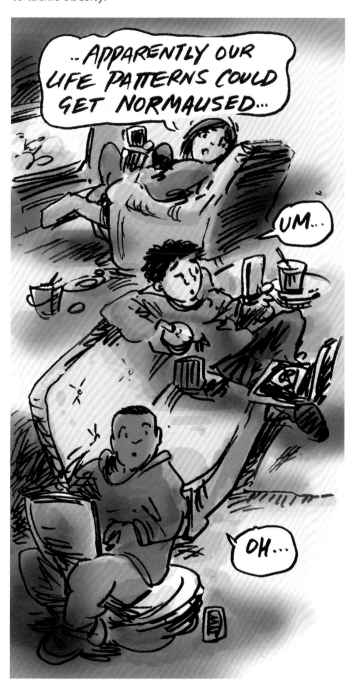

The research, published in the *International Journal of Environmental Research and Public Health,* found that among 400 randomly-selected college students from two FE institutions in southern England, more than 90% said that they failed to meet nationally recommended exercise targets, with three in ten not doing any exercise at all.

The survey was conducted by researchers at the University of Reading in partnership with further education colleges in Farnborough and Kent, and took a random sample of students to look at various factors associated with health and obesity.

Lead researcher Sunbal Naureen Bhatti from the School of Biological Sciences at the University of Reading said:

'This paper provides a picture of what 16-18 year olds are choosing to do with their health at a key transitional phase between childhood and adulthood. This is an important stage in life, as patterns of behaviour may become normalised, leading to obesity in later life.

'Although only one in five participants had a BMI that classified them as obese, we see several concerning factors that may lead to longer-term obesity. In particular, very few participants said that they were engaging in anything close to the recommended amount of exercise, and only one in five were eating the recommended "five a day" intake of fruit and veg.'

The study also shows how gender norms may be influencing participation in exercise and attitudes towards exercise at a formative time.

Only 7% of female students surveyed said that they were meeting the guidelines on exercise, and 64% said that they were 'unfit'. Meanwhile, 55% of males surveyed said that they were fit, but nearly a quarter did no exercise at all, with 86% failing to meet recommended guidelines.

Bhatti said:

'Taken together, the behaviours that we see in this sample of college students is something that we should be concerned about. The vast majority of participants cited "no time" or "don't want to" when asked why they didn't meet exercise targets, and yet we saw a strong association between lack of exercise and engaging in screen time either computing, gaming or watching TV.

'We recognise that this is a small study carried out in only two colleges, but we think there are important wider lessons here for public health, particularly as the UK government launches its new strategy to tackle obesity. To successfully make long-term efforts to tackle obesity in the UK, we must consider this age group as critical, when young people are beginning to exert more independence over their lifestyle.'

11 August 2020

Key Facts

- Worldwide obesity has nearly tripled since 1975. (page 1)
- In 2016, more than 1.9 billion adults, 18 years and older, were overweight. Of these over 650 million were obese. (page 1)
- 39% of adults aged 18 years and over were overweight in 2016, and 13% were obese. (page 1)
- Most of the world's population live in countries where overweight and obesity kills more people than underweight. (page 1)
- 38 million children under the age of 5 were overweight or obese in 2019. (page 1)
- Over 340 million children and adolescents aged 5-19 were overweight or obese in 2016. (page 1)
- 47% of children and young people were meeting the current physical activity guidelines. (page 6)
- 4% of primary school age children severely obese in Greece, Italy, Spain and San Marino. (page 9)
- Higher rates of maternal education were another factor that reduced the risk of severe obesity. (page 10)
- Almost 7 out of 10 men, and 6 out of 10 women in England are overweight or living with obesity. (page 11) children not eating a healthy diet will not perform as well at school as those who are well nourished. (page 13)
- Research found children aged between five and 17 should spend an hour a day doing moderate to vigorous exercise and no more than two hours a day in front of a screen. (page 14)
- More than three-quarters of teenagers spend more than two hours a day interacting with screens. (page 14)
- Four out of five teenagers in the UK are not doing enough exercise. (page 15)
- Boys in the Philippines (93 per cent) and girls in South Korea (97 per cent) were found to be the most inactive. (page 15)
- Men (70%) were more likely to be active than women (65%). (page 16)
- 47% of children and young people are meeting the current guidelines of taking part in sport and physical activity for an average of 60 minutes or more every day. (page 17)
- 35% of children in the least affluent families do fewer than 30 minutes of activity a day, compared to 22% of children from the most affluent families. (page 17)
- Around one-third of kids have a weight classed as overweight or obese before they even leave primary school. (page 19)
- Our activity levels are around 20% lower than in the 1960s. (page 19)
- Across most countries, women are less active than men (global average of 31·7% for inactive women vs 23·4% for inactive men). (page 26)
- Girls aged 3–11 years experienced less enjoyment from being physically active and less confidence in their sporting ability than boys as they got older. (page 26)
- Women were found to be more anxious about going out to exercise, more affected by caring responsibilities, comparatively worse off financially and more affected by the reduction in group activities such as exercise classes. (page 27)
- 70 per cent of women do say that it is 'more important than ever to be active'. (page 28)
- Pupils are being taught fewer hours of PE than they were a decade ago. (page 30)
- 80 per cent were failing to do the 60 minutes of daily physical exercise recommended by the chief medical officer. (page 30)
- One in four schools have reduced PE's presence on the timetable since 2017. (page 30)
- 42 per cent of teenage girls meet physical activity guidelines and just under a third of girls (32 per cent) are inactive, engaging in less than an average of 30 minutes' activity per day. (page 33)
- 32 per cent of women said that they couldn't prioritise exercise during lockdown as they had too much to do for others. (page 33
- 65 per cent of men are likely to be active, in comparison to 61 per cent of women. (page 33)
- 92% of school staff believe being physically active helps with school work, and 91% of students report feeling that physical activity can improve their mental and physical health. (page 35)
- Active students are happier (70% vs 50%) and more confident to try sport (76% vs 38%) than inactive students. (page 35)
- 87% of staff feel that being physically active has a positive impact on the school environment (ethos, values, culture, identity). (page 35)
- Teenagers spent about an hour and a half (93 minutes) longer each day sitting still or lying down at age 16 compared to age 12. (page 37)
- About 17% to 18% of teenagers had symptom scores that might mean they had depression at age 18. (page 37)
- In 2015, 42% of 14-year-old girls and boys said they currently were trying to lose weight, compared to 30% in 2005. (page 38)
- Both girls and boys also became more likely to over-estimate their weight from 1986 to 2005, and even more so by 2015. (page 38)
- Only one in five participants had a BMI classified as obese - but nine out of ten 16-18 year olds admit not exercising enough. (page 39)
- Three in ten did no exercise per week. (page 39)
- Eight out of ten not eating enough fruit and veg, with one in ten eating no fruit or veg at all, and half only eating 1-2 portions a day. (page 39)

BMI (body mass index)

An abbreviation which stands for 'body mass index' and is used to determine whether an individual's weight is in proportion to their height. If a person's BMI is below 18.5 they are usually seen as being underweight. If a person has a BMI greater than or equal to 25 they are classed as overweight, and a BMI of 30 and over is obese. As BMI is the same for both sexes and adults of all ages, it provides the most useful population-level measure of overweight and obesity. However, it should be considered a rough guide because it may not correspond to the same degree of 'fatness' in different individuals (e.g. a body builder could have a BMI of 30 but would not be obese because his weight would be primarily muscle rather than fat).

Diet

The variety of food and drink that someone eats on a regular basis. The phrase 'on a diet' is also often used to refer to a period of controlling what one eats while trying to lose weight.

Exercise

Physical activity that helps to improve and maintain a healthy body and mind. Exercise can be as easy as walking, swimming or dancing, to more intensive activity such as weight training, aerobics or High-Intensity Interval Training (HIIT).

Exercise intensity

This refers to how hard you exercise. Exercise intensity can be broken down into light, moderate or vigorous. Light exercise intensity feels easy; you have no noticeable changes in your breathing pattern and don't break a sweat. Moderate exercise intensity feels somewhat hard; your breath quickens and you develop a sweat after about ten minutes of activity (e.g. leisurely cycling, brisk walk, gardening). Vigorous exercise intensity feels very challenging; you can't carry on a conversation due to deep, rapid breathing and you develop a sweat after a few minutes of activity (e.g. jumping rope, basketball, running).

Fitness

The condition of being physically healthy (e.g. described as being in shape). Remember, fitness can also apply to our mental health and well-being. A high level of fitness is usually the result of regular exercise and a proper nutrition regime.

Fitness tracker

A wearable device that monitors fitness levels. Many of these devices track steps, heart rate, stairs climbed, sleep patterns, etc.

HIIT (High Intensity Interval Training)

Short bursts of high intensity exercise designed to increase the heart rate. Said to be particularly good for burning fat.

Inclusive sport

Sport which is inclusive does not discriminate on the grounds of gender, ethnicity, sexual orientation or disability. Sport is usually segregated where athletes have a physical difference which makes equal competition difficult – men and women do not generally compete against each other, for example, nor disabled and able-bodied athletes. This is called classification. However, there is no ban on any athlete competing in a separate competition. This is why the term 'sport equity' is sometimes used rather than equality. Athletes should be protected from discrimination and unfair treatment, such as racist and homophobic chanting at football matches.

Malnutrition

Malnutrition essentially means 'poor nutrition'. There are two types of malnutrition: undernutrition (when a person's diet is lacking in nutrients and sustenance they need) and overnutrition (when a person's diet is getting far too many nutrients for the body to cope with). Malnutrition can affect anybody, although it tends to be more common in developing countries where there are shortages of food.

Nutrition

The provision of materials needed by the body for growth, maintenance and sustaining life. Commonly when people talk about nutrition, they are referring to the healthy and balanced diet we all need to eat in order for the body to function properly.

Obesity

When someone is overweight to the extent that their BMI is 30 or above, they are classed as obese. Obesity is increasing in the UK and is associated with a number of health problems, such as an increased risk of heart disease and type 2 diabetes. Worldwide obesity has more than doubled since 1980 and this is most likely due to our more sedentary lifestyle, combined with a lack of physical exercise.

Overweight

A body weight that is greater than what is considered to normal or healthy in relation to height. An overweight person BMI would be between 25 and 29.9. This does not, however, mean that an overweight person is fat – people who are muscular can have a higher BMI without much fat.

Physical activity

Physical activity includes all forms of activity, such as walking or cycling, active play, work-related activity, active recreation such as working out in a gym, dancing, gardening or competitive sport like football. Regular physical activity can reduce the risk of many chronic health conditions including coronary heart disease, type 2 diabetes, cancer and obesity. Regular physical activity also has positive benefits for mental health as it can reduce anxiety and enhance moods and self-esteem, which reduces the risk of depression.

Activities

Brainstorming

♦ What is fitness?

♦ How much exercise should you be doing each day, based on your age?

♦ What activities can be good exercise?

♦ What is BMI?

♦ What does the term 'overweight' mean?

♦ What does the term 'obesity' mean?

Research

♦ Research how much activity you should be doing per week, based on your age. Create an exercise plan that you believe would be easy to integrate into your daily routine. For example, getting off the bus one stop early and walking the rest of the way, playing sport after school, doing an exercise class or following an exercise DVD at home.

♦ Talk to some friends and relatives about their experiences of PE at school. Think of at least five questions to ask and make a note of the respondent's age and gender. Include graphs to illustrate the difference between male and female experiences of PE.

♦ Research a new sport or fitness activity that you have always wanted to know more about. Find out how popular the activity is and how many people participate. Create a factsheet about the sport/activity.

♦ Do some research on the link between exercise and mental health – do they complement each other? Create a questionnaire and ask friends and family if they think that exercise is good for both mind and body.

♦ In small groups, discuss the sports or activities you enjoy doing. Make notes on what makes exercise enjoyable, and on reasons why people may not enjoy exercise.

♦ Do some research on malnutrition. Is it possible to be a healthy weight, but also be malnourished? Can you be overweight when you are eating nutritious foods?

♦ In pairs, look at the link between nutrition and exercise. How can a healthy diet, combined with physical activity, benefit you?

♦ In small groups, list all the sports/activities you can think of. Are any of these activities stereotypically male or female, or are they neutral? Sort the activities into these groups and then think of ways you can promote these for everyone to enjoy.

Design

♦ Choose one of the articles from this book and create an illustration that highlights its key message.

♦ Design a leaflet explaining obesity and its causes.

♦ Design a timetable of activities that can fit in with a daily routine of either; a child, young adult or elderly person.

♦ Create a poster to promote a sport/activity of your choice and make sure you include its benefits.

♦ Create an idea for an app that will help people find easy ways to keep active.

♦ Choose one of the articles in this book and create an infograph with the key themes of that article.

Oral

♦ Choose one of the illustrations from this book and, in pairs, discuss what you think the artist was trying to portray with their image.

♦ In pairs, create a presentation aimed at people over 60 explaining the benefits of exercise and suggesting ways they can stay active.

♦ In small groups, discuss why you think some people are less likely to meet the NHS exercise guidelines. Share with the rest of your class.

♦ Do you think it is appropriate for young children to be weighed at school, and for letters to be sent to their parents if they are considered at risk of being overweight? Debate this as a class.

♦ In small groups, discuss ways that you can keep active for free. Consider different age groups and activities that may suit them better.

♦ In pairs, discuss reasons why people may avoid exercise.

Reading/Writing

♦ Write a short summary of one of the articles in this book. Highlight the three key points.

♦ Imagine you work for a company that manufactures 'wearable technology'. Your company has released a new fitness tracker watch, aimed at young people, and wants to try and sell it in bulk to local schools. Write a letter to the head teacher of a local school, explaining why you think it would benefit their pupils to wear a fitness tracker and why he/she should invest in them.

♦ Write a letter to the head of the PE department with your thoughts on your PE lessons and how they could be improved. You could use feedback from the survey that you created, or use your own ideas.

♦ Write a blog post on a physical activity that you enjoy.

♦ Read the article 'Dieting and weight worries on rise in teens'. Imagine you have body worries, write a letter to an agony aunt/uncle and then write their reply.

Acknowledgements

The publisher is grateful for permission to reproduce the material in this book. While every care has been taken to trace and acknowledge copyright, the publisher tenders its apology for any accidental infringement or where copyright has proved untraceable. The publisher would be pleased to come to a suitable arrangement in any such case with the rightful owner.

The material reproduced in *ISSUES* books is provided as an educational resource only. The views, opinions and information contained within reprinted material in *ISSUES* books do not necessarily represent those of Independence Educational Publishers and its employees.

Images

Cover image courtesy of iStock. All other images courtesy of Pixabay and Unsplash, except pages 1: Rawpixel, 2: Freepik-jcomp, 13: Freepik

Icons

Icons on pages 18, 21 & 34 were made by Freepik from www.flaticon.com.

Illustrations

Simon Kneebone: pages 23, 33 & 39.

Angelo Madrid: pages 2, 26 & 36.

Additional acknowledgements

The press release reproduced on page 39 refers to the following research publication: : Bhatti, S.N., Watkin, E., Butterfill, J., & Li, J-M. (2020) 'Recognition of 16–18 year old adolescents for guiding physical activity interventions: A cross-sectional study' *International Journal of Environmental Research and Public Health* (Section: Exercise and Health), 17(14), pp. 5002. https://doi.org/10.3390/ijerph17145002

With thanks to the Independence team: Shelley Baldry, Danielle Lobban, Jackie Staines and Jan Sunderland.

Tracy Biram

Cambridge, January 2021